The Short Textbook of
MEDICAL LABORATORY
for Technicians

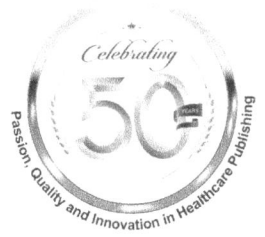

The Short Textbook of
MEDICAL LABORATORY
for Technicians

Third Edition

Satish Gupte MD
Professor
Department of Microbiology
Kathmandu Medical College
Kathmandu, Nepal

Ex-Professor and Head
Department of Microbiology
Gian Sagar Medical College and Hospital
Patiala, Punjab, India

Ex-Professor and Head
Department of Microbiology
Adesh Institute of Medical Sciences and Research Center
Bhatinda, Punjab, India
and
Government Medical College
Jammu, Jammu and Kashmir, India

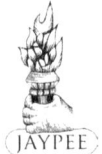

JAYPEE BROTHERS MEDICAL PUBLISHERS
The Health Sciences Publisher
New Delhi | London

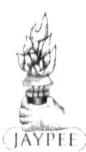 **Jaypee Brothers Medical Publishers (P) Ltd**

Headquarters
Jaypee Brothers Medical Publishers (P) Ltd
EMCA House
23/23-B, Ansari Road, Daryaganj
New Delhi - 110 002, India
Landline: +91-11-23272143, +91-11-23272703
+91-11-23282021, +91-11-23245672
Email: jaypee@jaypeebrothers.com

Corporate Office
Jaypee Brothers Medical Publishers (P) Ltd
4838/24, Ansari Road, Daryaganj
New Delhi 110 002, India
Phone: +91-11-43574357
Fax: +91-11-43574314
Email: jaypee@jaypeebrothers.com

Overseas Office
J.P. Medical Ltd
83 Victoria Street, London
SW1H 0HW (UK)
Phone: +44 20 3170 8910
Fax: +44 (0)20 3008 6180
Email: info@jpmedpub.com

Website: www.jaypeebrothers.com
Website: www.jaypeedigital.com

© 2021, Managing Editor: Mrs Jyotsna Gupte and Jaypee Brothers Medical Publishers

The views and opinions expressed in this book are solely those of the original contributor(s)/author(s) and do not necessarily represent those of editor(s) of the book.

All rights reserved. No part of this publication may be reproduced, stored or transmitted in any form or by any means, electronic, mechanical, photocopying, recording or otherwise, without the prior permission in writing of the publishers.

All brand names and product names used in this book are trade names, service marks, trademarks or registered trademarks of their respective owners. The publisher is not associated with any product or vendor mentioned in this book.

Medical knowledge and practice change constantly. This book is designed to provide accurate, authoritative information about the subject matter in question. However, readers are advised to check the most current information available on procedures included and check information from the manufacturer of each product to be administered, to verify the recommended dose, formula, method and duration of administration, adverse effects and contraindications. It is the responsibility of the practitioner to take all appropriate safety precautions. Neither the publisher nor the author(s)/editor(s) assume any liability for any injury and/or damage to persons or property arising from or related to use of material in this book.

This book is sold on the understanding that the publisher is not engaged in providing professional medical services. If such advice or services are required, the services of a competent medical professional should be sought.

Every effort has been made where necessary to contact holders of copyright to obtain permission to reproduce copyright material. If any have been inadvertently overlooked, the publisher will be pleased to make the necessary arrangements at the first opportunity. The **CD/DVD-ROM** (if any) provided in the sealed envelope with this book is complimentary and free of cost. **Not meant for sale.**

Inquiries for bulk sales may be solicited at: jaypee@jaypeebrothers.com

The Short Textbook of Medical Laboratory for Technicians

First Edition: 1998
 Reprint: 2004
Second Edition: 2014
Third Edition: **2021**

ISBN : 978-93-90595-04-4

Printed at

Dedicated to
*Loving memory of
my parents*

Preface to the Third Edition

The Short Textbook of Medical Laboratory for Technicians happens to tackle all specialties of clinical laboratory, such as microbiology, biochemistry, blood transfusion and pathology (cytology, histopathology, hematology). Many times many books are required to clarify simple and minor queries that this book readily provide. Overwhelming response has encouraged me to bring out this third edition of *The Short Textbook of Medical Laboratory for Technicians*.

It is worthwhile to mention that techniques are discussed step by step, briefly in a very simple and understandable language on microbiology, hematology, immunology, cytology, mycology, parasitology, bacteriology and clinical aspects. New material, such as phase contrast microscope, dark field microscope, interference microscope, polarizing microscope, polarization microscope, electron microscope, PCR technique, gas chromatography, BACTEC, automation in clinical laboratory and clinical cytology is added.

Dr DS Jamwal, Ex-Professor and Head, Department of Biochemistry, Government Medical College, Jammu, Jammu and Kashmir, India covered biochemistry in easy and understandable manner. At the same time, there is decorated latest updated addition of clinical biochemical techniques from Mr Naveen Shrivastava, Department of Biochemistry, Kathmandu Medical College, Kathmandu, Nepal. Also there is another contribution on automation in clinical biochemistry. The contribution of these eminent biochemists has definitely enhanced the utility of this volume.

Shri Jitendar P Vij (Group Chairman), Mr Ankit Vij (Managing Director), Mr MS Mani (Group President), Dr Madhu Choudhary (Publishing Head–Education), Ms Pooja Bhandari (Production Head), Ms Sunita Katla (Executive Assistant to Group Chairman and Publishing Manager), Ms Samina Khan (Executive Assistant to Publishing Head–Education), Dr Akanksha Singh (Development Editor), Mr Rajesh Sharma (Production Coordinator), Ms Seema Dogra (Cover Visualizer), Mr Vakil Khan (Proofreader), Mr Akshay Thakur (Typesetter), Mr Sanjeev Kumar (Graphic Designer), and expert team of M/s Jaypee Brothers Medical Publishers (P) Ltd, New Delhi, India, have worked hard to bring out this book in excellent and impressive form. I am grateful to all of them.

I am also thankful to Faculty, Department of Microbiology, Kathmandu Medical College, Kathmandu, Nepal and also to my postgraduates Dr Anjita and Dr Sita, for their typing and editing.

The manuscript of third edition would not have been available without the best wishes and moral support of my wife Mrs Jyotsna Gupte (Managing Editor of this book) and my son Anubhav Gupte. I am highly obliged to them.

I wish this edition of the book *The Short Textbook of Medical Laboratory for Technicians* has healthy criticism and suggestions for improvement of upcoming editions.

Satish Gupte

Preface to the First Edition

An ideal laboratory technician is expected to be in possession of sound knowledge of procedures and test techniques. It is generally seen that sometimes many books are required for obtaining answers of simple and minor queries.

These problems and many others are taken care of in this volume *The Short Textbook of Medical Laboratory for Technicians*. The techniques are discussed briefly and in simple and easy-to-understand language on microbiology, hematology, immunology, histopathology, blood transfusion, clinical pathology and clinical biochemistry. These are compiled under headings: name of technique, principle, requirements, procedure, and results-cum-interpretation. The introductory chapters make the book more useful to average laboratory workers.

Dr DS Jamwal, Assistant Professor, Department of Biochemistry, Government Medical College, Jammu, Jammu and Kashmir, India, has been kind enough to contribute the section, *Clinical Biochemistry* and allied topics. His expertise, contribution and constructive criticism are bound to enhance the utility of the book.

I express my sincere thanks to Dr Vijay Sharma, for going through the manuscript and for valuable suggestions.

It is my privilege to express gratitude to my wife Mrs Jyotsna Gupte, and son, master Anubhav Gupte, for extending full cooperation and help in the preparation of the book.

Well-deserving thanks is extended to M/s Jaypee Brothers Medical Publishers (P) Ltd, New Delhi, India, for bringing out the book in a very impressive form.

Hopefully, the book will find wide acceptance by all concerned and laboratory technicians in particular. Comments and criticism for the improvement of future edition are most welcome.

Satish Gupte

Contents

Section 1: Medical Laboratory

1. **General Introduction**   3
   Guidelines   3
   - Code of Ethics for Laboratory Technicians   3
   - Responsibilities of Medical Technician   3
   - Instructions for Laboratory Technicians   5
   - Arrangement of Laboratory   6
   - Disposal of Laboratory Infected Material and Clinical Specimens   13
   - Reagents and their Preparation   15
   - Indicator   23
   - Preparation of Solutions in General   24
   - Dilutions of Sample or Solution   26

2. **Laboratory Equipment**   29
   - Microscope   29
   - Phase Contrast Microscopy   35
   - Dark Ground Microscope   36
   - Polarizing Microscope   37
   - Electron Microscope   38
   - Interference Microscope   39
   - Photometer or Colorimeter   40
   - Autoclave   42
   - Biological Safety Cabinet   43
   - Types of Safety Cabinets   43
   - Hot Air Oven   47
   - Centrifuge Machine   48
   - Other Types of Centrifuge Machine   50
   - Balance   50
   - Autoanalyzer   53
   - Inspissator   56
   - Wood's Lamp   57
   - Water Bath   59
   - Distillation Plant   61
   - Polymerase Chain Reaction   62

- Principle 62
- Component of PCR 63
- Results 64
- Types of PCR 64
- Multiples PCR 65
- Nested PCR 65

Section 2: Human Body Fluids

3. Body Fluids 69

Examination of Urine 69
- Collection of Urine 69
- Esbach's Albuminometer 70
- Routine Examination of Urine 71
- Urinometer 72

Examination of Cerebrospinal Fluid 81
- Functions of CSF 81
- Features of CSF 82
- Collection of Specimen 82
- Silver Nitrate Titration Method 84

Stool Examination 86
- Collection of Stool 86

Examination of Sputum 89
- Collection of Sputum Specimen 89

Examination of Semen 93
- Collection of Semen 93

Section 3: Microbiology

4. Microbiology 99

Bacteriology 99
- Microbiology 99
- Morphology and Examination of Bacteria 102
- Demonstration of Bacteria in Unstained Preparations 104
- Demonstration of Bacteria in Stained Preparation 105
- Sterilization 108

- Disinfection of Important Articles *109*
- Urinals *110*
- Bedding *110*
- Mattresses *110*
- Blood Spill *110*
- Blood Stained Linen *111*
- Bowls *111*
- Cheatle Forceps *111*
- Thermometers *111*
- Buckets *111*
- Catheter *111*
- Cytoscope *112*
- Endoscope *112*
- Culturing of Bacteria *112*
- Culture Media *112*
- Solid Media *114*
- Culture Methods *117*
- Biochemical Test *118*
- Brief Description of Some Bacteria *121*
- Pneumococci *122*
- Gonococci *122*
- *Clostridium tetani* *122*
- Tubercle Bacilli (*Mycobacterium tuberculosis*) *123*
- Diphtheria Bacilli *123*
- *Salmonella typhi* *124*
- *Vibrio cholerae* (Cholera Bacilli) *124*
- *Treponema pallidum* *125*
- Bacteriological Examination of Water *125*

Mycology *127*
- Methods for Studying Fungi in Specimen *127*

Parasitology *129*
- Protozoa *129*
- Malarial Parasites *131*
- Helminths *132*

Immunology *135*
- Widal Test *136*
- Latex Fixation Test for Rheumatoid Factor *137*
- C-Reactive Protein *138*
- Latex ASO (Antistreptolysin-O) *139*
- Pregnancy Test (Gravindex Test) *140*

- Venereal Disease Research Laboratory Test   140
- Kahn's Test   141
- ELISA Test   142
- Results   144

Section 4: Hematology

5. Hematology   147
- Plasma   147
- Red Blood Cells (Erythrocytes)   148
- White Blood Cells (Leukocytes)   148
- Platelets (Thrombocytes)   148
- Estimation of Hemoglobin   149

Normal Range of Hemoglobin   155
- Total Red Blood Cell Count   155
- Erythrocyte Sedimentation Rate   158
- Packed Cell Volume   161
- Absolute Values and Color Index   162
- Total Leukocyte Count   164
- Differential Leukocyte Count   166
- Reticulocyte Count   170
- Absolute Eosinophil Count   171
- Platelet Count   172
- Coagulation Time   173
- Bleeding Time (Duke's Method)   175
- Collection of Blood   175
- Anticoagulants   177
- Lupus Erythematosus Cell Phenomenon   178
- Fragility of Red Blood Cells for Hemolytic Disorders   178
- Prothrombin Time   179
- Clot Retraction   180
- Bone Marrow Examination   180

Section 5: Blood Transfusion

6. Preservation of Blood   185
- Organization of Blood Bank   185
- Blood Transfusion   186

- Selection of Blood Donors *189*
- Collection of Blood *189*
- Cross-matching of Blood *190*

Section 6: Histopathology

7. Histopathology — 195
- Histopathological Examination *195*
- Histopathological Techniques *196*
- Museum Techniques *201*
- Fine Needle Aspiration Cytology *202*
- Smear Preparation *204*
- Frozen Section *207*
- Fixation *207*
- Staining Technique for Rapid Diagnosis *208*
- Exfoliative Cytology *209*
- Special Staining Methods *209*
- Stain for Amyloid *210*
- Stain for Hemosiderin (Perls Stain) *210*
- Wilder's Silver Impregnation Method (Reticulum Fibers) *210*
- Staining for Fat *211*
- Verhoeff's Elastic Stain *212*

Section 7: Biochemistry

8. Biochemistry — 215
- Estimation of Blood Glucose *215*
- Other Methods for Estimation of Blood Glucose Levels *217*
- Glucose Tolerance Test *218*
- Blood Urea Estimation *220*
- Other Methods *222*
- Blood Creatinine Estimation *222*
- Estimation of Total Proteins and Albumin in Blood *224*
- Albumin *225*
- Blood Cholesterol Estimation *227*
- Serum Bilirubin *228*
- Estimation of Serum Uric Acid *230*
- Estimation of Serum Alkaline Phosphatase *232*
- Estimation of Serum Acid Phosphatase *234*
- Estimation of Serum Amylase *235*
- Automation in Clinical Laboratory *240*

Appendices   247

Appendix 1   247
- Hematological Values   247
- Biochemical Values   249

Appendix 2   252
- Electron Microscope   252
- Working Principle of TEM   254

Appendix 3   258
- Protocol for Conducting COVID-19 PCR   258
- Reagent Preparation of High Pure NA Kit   258
- RT-PCR Protocol   260

Appendix 4   262
- Bactec   262
- VITEK 2 Compact System   264

Index   267

SECTION 1

Medical Laboratory

Section Outline
- ❖ General Introduction
- ❖ Laboratory Equipment

CHAPTER 1

General Introduction

GUIDELINES

Code of Ethics for Laboratory Technicians

Following ethics are expected to be followed by laboratory technicians:
- No assumption or guess work without proper tests of a specimen as per standard methods.
- Accuracy and correctness in test reports should be observed.
- Exhaustive standard method to ascertain correct report in given analysis.
- Never postpone the work.
- Laboratory report should only be sent to the doctor concerned. They are not to be disclosed or discussed with patients or attendants of patients.
- Strictly follow the instruction of doctors and report only the tests they require.

Responsibilities of Medical Technician

General
- Keep the laboratory clean.
- Chemicals, equipment and glasswares should be kept at the places marked for them.
- Glassware and equipment should be neat and clean.
- Properly label the chemicals' bottles and reagents with the name.
- Handle the microscope with care.
- Clean and sterilize the material as required.
- Dispose off the specimens and infected material in a safer manner.
- Handle and process the specimens observing all safety measures.
- Maintenance of records of laboratory tests done and preparation of monthly report.

Section 1: Medical Laboratory

- Indent for supplies to the laboratory through medical officer and make proper enteries to register (consumable items/stock items). Also ensure the safe storage and utilization of material/items received.

Laboratory Investigations

- For examination of urine, do as under:
  - Test specific gravity and pH
  - Test for sugar
  - Test for protein (albumin)
  - Test for bile pigments and bile salts
  - Test for ketone bodies
  - Microscopic examination.
- For stool examination:
  - Naked eye examination
  - Microscopic examination.
- Examination of blood may be done as under:
  - Collection of blood specimen by finger-prick technique
  - Hemoglobin estimation
  - RBC count
  - WBC count (total and differential)
  - Preparation, staining and examination of thick and thin blood smears for malarial parasites, microfilariae, etc.
  - Erythrocytic sedimentation rate (ESR).
- Sputum examination can be carried out by:
  - Preparation, staining and examination of sputum smear for *Mycobacterium tuberculosis* or fungi
  - Culture the specimen when required.
- Carry out examination of skin and nasal smear:
  - Preparation, staining and examination of skin/nasal/earlobe smear for *Mycobacterium leprae*, fungi, etc.
- Perform examination of the semen:
  - Naked eye examination
  - Sperm count and motility with the help of microscope.
- Prepare throat and pus swabs, wherever indicated.
- Preparation of media and to do tests for identification of bacteria.
- In mycology, laboratory to prepare Potassium hydroxide (KOH) preparation and put up specimen on Sabouraud's medium.
- To work in immunology or serology laboratory for performing tests like Widal, pregnancy, C-reactive protein (CRP), etc.

- In histopathology laboratory,
  - Naked eye examination of specimen
  - Processing of tissue
  - Cutting sections.
- In blood bank to do grouping cross-matching, collection and storage of blood from donors.
- To work in biochemistry for various tests like blood sugar, blood cholesterol, blood urea, etc.

Instructions for Laboratory Technicians

- Always wear apron before entering the laboratory to prevent contamination of the clothes and to avoid catching and carrying infection
- Place the well-being and service to the sick as first priority
- Be loyal to laboratory work and keep high standard of work
- Respect and work in harmony with your colleagues and be courteous and considerate to the attendants of the patient
- Never smoke, drink or dine within laboratory
- Keep laboratory neat and clean
- Arrange the laboratory in such a way that each article is placed at proper place. Always place the chemicals and other articles at the same place after use
- Handle specimen with care. Wash your hands thoroughly with soap and water and rinse them with disinfectant solution after carrying out the tests
- Avoid using pipette by mouth. Use rubber bulb teats on the pipette to suck up the material
- Never use refrigerator in the laboratory for storing edibles, etc.
- After finishing work, swab the working table with a disinfectant solution. Make it a point that floor is swept and swabbed with disinfectant solution daily
- All contaminated liquid or solid material should be decontaminated and autoclaved or incinerated before disposal
- If infected material drops on the bench, pour phenol on it, soak it with clean paper and burn the paper or keep it in disinfectant for final disposal.
- Always take care of your health by taking proper balanced diet and regular exercise to avoid catching infection in the laboratory

- Workers must take vaccine against cholera, typhoid, hepatitis B, tetanus, tuberculosis, etc. Always keep your nails short and clean. One should wash hands with soap and water frequently.

Arrangement of Laboratory

An ideal laboratory (**Fig. 1.1**) should have adequate light which may be natural sunlight or electric light. It should be arranged in such a way so that it has:
- A space for collection of specimens plus records in the form of requisition slips and proper entry in the register, test reports on proper forms, etc.
- Refrigerator
- Sink, drain
- A space for staining
- A space where stool and urine examinations may be done
- A space where blood examination may be performed
- A space preferably near window should be reserved for keeping and using of microscope.

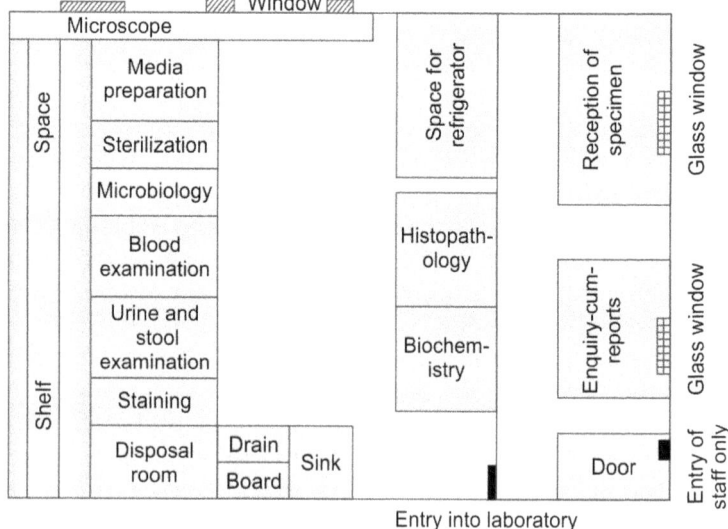

Fig. 1.1: Laboratory arrangement

Chapter 1: General Introduction

Main Requirements for Laboratory

Furniture

- Laboratory table unit having:
    - Formica top and knee space
    - Stainless steel sink with drain board
    - Storage cabinets fitted under the table
    - Reagent rack-fitted above laboratory table.
- Writing table
- Steel almirah
- Chair without arms
- Revolving chair
- Dustbin

Instruments

- Microscope
- Centrifuge machine
- Refrigerator
- Autoclave
- Sahli's hemoglobinometer (Complete)
- ESR stand and tubes
- Colorimeter
- Hot air oven
- Laminar flow
- Wireloops
- Spirit lamp
- Balance
- pH meter
- Incinerator
- Gas-pack jar and envelops
- Distillation plant
- Needles destroyer
- Colorimeter
- Sysmex cell counter.

Glassware

- Beakers
- Bottles
- Centrifuge tubes

Section 1: Medical Laboratory

- Coverslips
- Drop bottles
- Flasks
- Funnels
- Glass cylinder
- Glass rods
- Glass tubing
- Measuring cylinder
- Pipettes
- Reagent bottles
- Staining tray
- Wash bottles
- Watch glasses
- Petri dish
- Syringes
- Wet chamber

Chemicals

- Acetic acid, glacial
- Acetone
- Ammonia
- Basic fuchsin
- Distilled water
- Ethanol 95% (ethyl alcohol)
- Ether
- Hydrochloric acid
- Hydrogen peroxide
- Immersion oil
- Methylated spirit
- Methyl alcohol
- Petroleum jelly (vaseline)
- Sodium bicarbonate
- Sodium dichromate
- Sodium nitroprusside
- Sulfur powder
- Sulfuric acid
- Tincture benzoin
- Xylene
- Glass jars
- Lysol

Stationery

- Examination request form
- Registers
- Report forms
- Monthly report form
- Gum
- Labels for bottles
- Office files
- Pens or ballpoint pens
- Glass marking pencils
- Rubber bands
- Ruler
- Stapler
- Staples
- Thread/string
- Plain papers
- Paint brush
- Brown paper
- Adhesive tape
- Pins
- Notepad

Miscellaneous

- Aluminum containers with screw caps (for packing specimen tubes or bottles)
- Platinum wire
- Aprons
- Bottle cleaning brushes
- Cheatle's forceps
- Cork screw
- Forceps
- Hagedorn needle or lancet for taking capillary blood
- Loop holders
- Slides tray
- Scalpel
- Scissors
- Buckets
- Duster
- Scrubbing brush
- Slide box

Section 1: Medical Laboratory

- Soap dish
- Test tube holders
- Test tube racks
- Thermometer
- Towels
- Applicator (wooden)
- Cotton swab sticks
- Cotton wool
- Detergent (powder and liquid)
- Filter paper
- Matchbox
- Nylon thread
- Tongue depressor
- Wire basket
- Nailcutter

Cleaning of Glasswares

Glasswares should be cleaned in the laboratory. It is necessary to get correct results. Cleaning of glasswares is done as under:
- *Cleaning of new glasswares*
    - Mix 3 liters of water and 60 ml of concentrated hydrochloric acid in bucket or basin
    - Leave the new glasswares completely dipped in this solution for 24 hours
    - Rinse twice with water and once with distilled water
    - Dry
- *Cleaning of dirty glasswares*
    - Rinse the glasswares twice in cold or lukewarm water
    - Now put the glasswares in solution of water and cleaning agent like washing powder kept in a bowl
    - Brush the glasswares inside the container. Leave to soak for 2 hours
    - Remove the articles one by one and rinse under tap water
    - Now soak them in distilled water
    - Keep glasswares on the pegs of a wall draining rack or upside down in a wire basket and allow to dry
    - Plug the containers with non-absorb cotton wool.
- *Cleaning of glass pipettes*
    - Soon after use, pipette must be rinsed in the container
    - After rinsing, place the pipettes in large plastic cylinder or bowl full of water or disinfectant solution (2% phenol) for 24 hours

- Soak in soap and water solution, brush and leave to soak for 2 to 3 hours
- Remove pipette one by one and rinse thoroughly in tap water. Finally, rinse with distilled water. Leave the pipette to dry.
- *Cleaning of dirty glass slides*
  - Slides with immersion oil are cleaned one by one by rubbing with newspaper
  - Prepare soap and water solution and soak slides in it for 24 hours.
  - Take the slide out one by one with forceps. Rinse them separately under the tap. Soak them in a bowl of water for 30 minutes
  - Now wipe and dry the slides.
- *Cleaning of coverslip*
  - Soak in weak detergent solution (200 ml water + 3 ml detergent + 15 ml of bleaching powder) in a beaker
  - Keep them soaked for 2 to 3 hours
  - Rinse out the beaker with tap water at least 4 times
  - Give a final rinse with distilled water
  - Drain the coverslips by keeping them on to a pad of gauze
  - Dry them and keep coverslips in a small Petri dish.
- *Preparation of grease-free coverslips*
  - In a cylinder, mix 10 ml of 95% ethanol and 10 ml of ether
  - Pour this solution in a Petri dish
  - Place about 30 coverslips one by one in this solution
  - Shake and wait for 10 minutes
  - Bring out coverslips one by one and place in petri dish.
- *Cleaning of syringes and needles*
  - Remove the part of syringe (Plunger, barrel) (**Fig. 1.2**)
  - Fill the barrel with water and put plunger into barrel. Now force the water out through needle several times
  - Remove the needle and rinse the hub cavity.
- *Dichromate cleaning solution*
  - Dissolve 25 gm of potassium dichromate in 25 ml of water
  - Slowly add with stirring 50 ml of concentrated sulfuric acid
  - When cool, store this solution in stoppered bottle
  - Always add acid to water
  - Glasswares are immersed in this solution overnight
  - Bring out glassware one by one and rinse in running tap water.

Section 1: Medical Laboratory

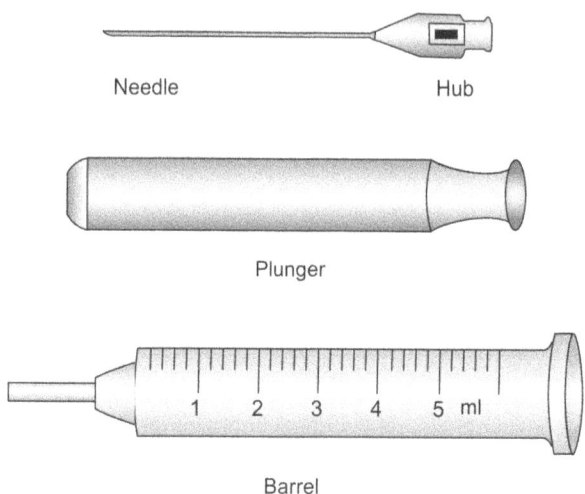

Fig. 1.2: Parts of syringe

White Apron

White apron is knee length apron worn by doctors and laboratory workers. It serves as barrier between doctor and patients. It is made up of white-colored cotton, linen or cotton polyesters, polyester blend. It can be washed at high temperature. The color of the apron is white because with white color, it is easy to perceive whether it is clean or not.

White apron was choosen because of following reason:
- Considered as a new standard of medical profession
- White color represents purity and goodness
- Conveys cleanliness
- White coat is considered as a garment of compassion
- White coat reminds doctors of their professional duties as prescribed by Hippocrates.

Uses of White Coat

- Faster recognition of doctors by patients
- White coats have large pockets to carry stethoscope
- Protection of clothes from being soiled
- Protection of self against contamination from surroundings and patients
- Helps in keeping body of doctors warm to some extent in winter.

Disposal of Laboratory Infected Material and Clinical Specimens

- Specimens like pus, urine, stool, etc. are usually full of disease causing germs
- After doing test, they must be destroyed properly
- Also germ-grown material, especially in microbiology laboratory, should be disposed of.

Following are the methods of disposal of germ containing objects:

Disposable Boxes Containing Stools, Urine, Sputum, etc.

Incineration

Construction of an incinerator (Fig. 1.3)
- It consists of leak proof drums
- Fix a strong metal grating about 1/3rd of the way up the drums
- Cut a wide opening or vent below the level of grating
- Adjust a removable lid for the drum.

Operating of incinerator
- At the end of each morning and afternoon's work, place all used stool, sputum, discarded culture material, etc. on the grating of incinerator
- All material should be kept in disposable cardboard cartons or other disposable boxes along with disinfectants like lysol
- Now close the metal drum tightly both lid and vent
- At the time of incineration, lid and vent should be kept opened
- Fill the bottom of the incinerator with sticks, paper, wood, coal, etc.

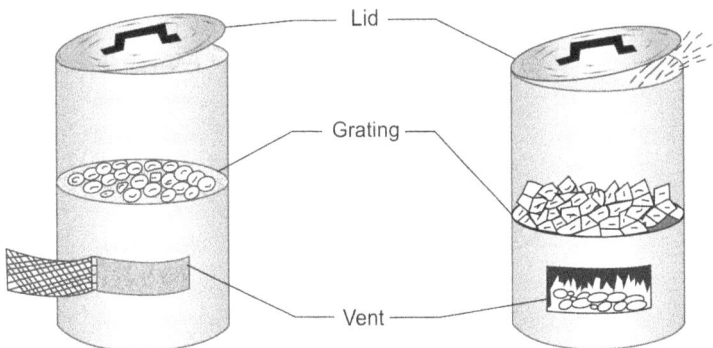

Fig. 1.3: Incinerator

Section 1: Medical Laboratory

- Keep the lid open and lit the fire. Keep the fire burning till germ containing material is completely burnt to ashes
- The ash so produced is not harmful and can be thrown on the refuse heap.

Burial of Germ Containing Material

- Dig a pit 4 to 5 meters deep and 1 to 2 meters wide in a corner of open piece of land
- Make a lid that fits tightly over the pit
- Upper rim of pit should be strengthened by lining it with bricks and stones
- Throw clinical germ containing specimens after doing tests into the pit. Replace the lid immediately (**Fig. 1.4**)
- At least once in a week cover the refuse with layer of 10 cm of dried leaves
- It is always better to use a layer of calcium carbonate instead of leaves.

Sterilization and Cleaning of Glass Containers Used for Germ Containing Materials

- Use disinfectant like Lysol (5%). Keep disinfectant for 24 hours in the container. Clean container with detergent like soap and water.

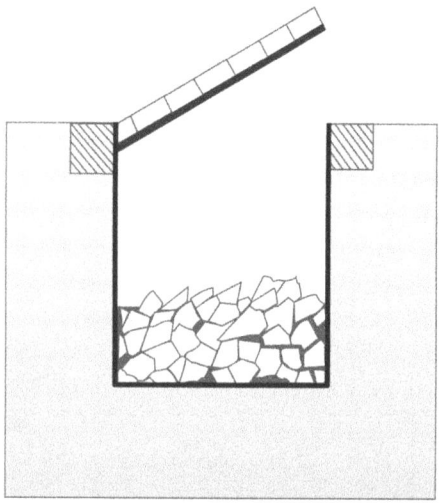

Fig. 1.4: Burial of germ containing material

Chapter 1: General Introduction

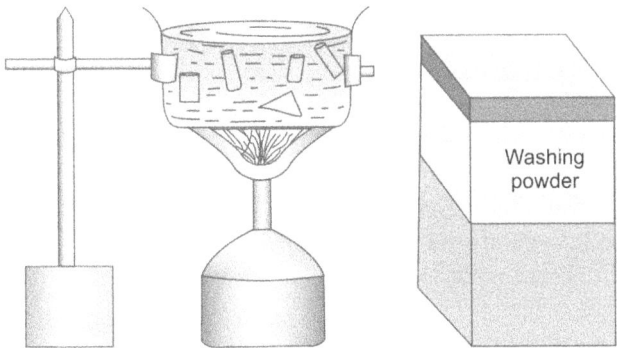

Fig. 1.5: Sterilization by boiling

- Autoclave the containers for 20 to 30 minutes at 120°C at 15 lbs pressure per square inch. Cool the container and clean jars with water and soap.
  i. Boil the container with detergent for 30 minutes in watering washing powder in strong solution (60 ml per liter of water) (**Fig. 1.5**).
  ii. Alternatively, water containing sodium carbonate crystal may be used.
- Container like tubes may be kept in 10% bleaching powder or 2% phenol for 24 hours. Rinse with water and then wash with soap and water.
- Tubes or bottles containing fresh blood may be rinsed in cold water and then kept in detergent solution.
- Tubes or bottles containing old blood for several days and weeks at room temperature and containing germs should be kept in 10% solution of commercial bleaching powder for 12 hours. Now rinse them with soap and water.

Reagents and Their Preparation

Acetic Acid 10% (100 gm/liter)

- Glacial acetic acid (CH_3COOH)   20 ml
- Distilled water   qs 200 ml

Acid Ethanol (For modified Ziehl-Neelsen Stain)

- Hydrochloric acid   3 ml
- Ethanol 70%   up to 100 ml

Barium Chloride 10% (100 gm/liter) Aqueous Solution

- Barium chloride ($BaCl_2$)   10 gm
- Distilled water   qs 100 ml

Benedict Qualitative Solution

- Copper sulphate ($CuSO_4.5H_2O$)   173.3 gm
- Trisodium citrate ($Na_3C_6H_5O_7.2H_2O$)   173.0 gm
- Sodium carbonate (Na_2CO_3) anhydrous   100.0 gm
- *Distilled water*:   1000 ml
  - Dissolve copper sulfate by heat in 100 ml water.
  - Dissolve the trisodium citrate and sodium carbonate in 800 ml of water.
  - Add the copper sulfate solution slowly to sodium carbonate/trisodium citrate solution, stirring constantly throughout.
  - Make up the total volume of solution as 1000 ml with distilled water.

Buffered Water (For Giemsa and Leishman Stains)

- Sodium hydrogen phosphate ($Na_2HPO_4.2H_2O$)   3.76 gm
- Potassium dihydrogen phosphate (KH_2PO_4) anhydrous   2.10 mg
- Distilled water   qs 1000 ml
  - Adjust pH of solution using narrow range pH paper   pH 7.0 to 7.2

Buffered Water (For JSB Stain)

- Disodium hydrogen phosphate   0.417 gm
- Potassium acid phosphate   0.752 gm
- Distilled water   2000 ml
- pH required   6.2 to 6.8

Carbol Fuchsin (For Ziehl-Neelsen Stain)

Solution A

- Saturated solution of basic fuchsin
  - Basic fuchsin   3 gm
  - Ethanol 95%   100 ml

Solution B

- Phenol solution 50 gm/liter (5%) aqueous
- Phenol   10 gm
- Distilled water   200 ml
  - Measure solution A   10 ml
  - Measure solution B   90 ml
  - Mix them and use carefully as it is highly poisonous

Carbol Fuchsin (For Modified Ziehl-Neelsen Stain)

- Basic fuchsin   5 gm
- Ethanol 95%   10 ml
- Phenol 5% solution   90 ml

Cary-Blair Transport (Holding) Medium

- Sodium thioglycolate   1.5 gm
- Disodium hydrogen phosphate (Na_3HPO_4) anhydrous   1.1 gm
- Sodium chloride   5.0 gm
- Agar   5.0 gm
- *Distilled water*:   991.0 ml
  - To be prepared in chemically clean glassware
  - Heat while mixing the contents till the solution becomes clear
  - Cool the mixture to 50°C
  - Add 9.0 ml of freshly prepared aqueous calcium chloride 1% (10 gm per liter)
  - Adjust pH to about 8.4
  - Pour 7.0 ml in properly rinsed and sterilized 9.0 ml screw-capped vials
  - Steam the vials containing media for 15 minutes, cool and tighten the cups.

Crystal Violet

Solution A

- Crystal violet   2.0 gm
- Ethanol 95%   20 ml

Solution B

- Ammonium oxalate [$(NH_4)C_2O_4 \cdot H_2O$]   0.8 gm

- Distilled water   80 ml
  - Mix solution A and B
  - Store for 24 hours before use
  - Filter through filter paper into staining bottle

Dichromate Cleaning Solution (For Cleaning Glasswares)

- Potassium dichromate ($K_2Cr_2O_7$)   100 gm
- Water   1000 ml
- Pure sulfuric acid   100 ml
  - Dissolve the dichromate in water
  - Add acid very carefully and slowly
  - Stirring should be continuous
  - Always remember that acid must be added to the water

EDTA (Dipotassium Salt Solution) 10%

- Dipotassium ethylene diamine tetra-acetate   20 gm
- Distilled water   qs 200 ml
  - For use pipette 0.04 ml of solution into a small clean container marked to hold 2.5 ml blood
  - Allow anticoagulant to dry by leaving the containers overnight on warm bench or in an incubator at 37°C.

Eosin (2%) Solution in Saline

- Eosin   2 gm
- Sodium chloride (0.85%) (8.5 gm/100 liter) in aqueous solution   qs 100 ml

Fouchet's Reagent

First prepare 10% solution of ferric chloride
- Ferric chloride $FeCl_3$ 10 gm
- Distilled water   qs 100 ml

Preparation of reagent
- Ferric chloride solution as prepared above   10 ml
- Trichloroacetic acid (CCl_3COOH)   25 gm
- Distilled water   100 ml
  - Dissolve trichloracetic acid in 70 ml of distilled water in volumetric flask

- Add 10 ml of the 10% ferric chloride solution
- Make the volume 100 ml with distilled water.

Giemsa Stain

- Powdered Giemsa stain   0.75 gm
- Methanol (CH_3OH)   65 ml
- Glycerol   35 ml
  - Put the ingredients in a bottle containing glass beads and shake
  - Shake the bottle 3 times a day for 4 consecutive days
  - Filter and use.

Gram Iodine Solution

- Iodine   3.3 gm
- Potassium iodide   6.6 gm
- Distilled water   100 ml
  - Measure 100 ml of water in cylinder.
  - First of all dissolve the potassium iodide in about 30 ml of the water
  - Now add iodine and mix until dissolved
  - Add the 70 ml water and mix well
  - Store in a brown bottle.

Hydrochloric Acid (0.1N) 0.1 mol/liter

- Hydrochloric acid (HCl) concentrated   8.6 ml
- Distilled water   qs 1000 ml
  - Measure 500 ml of water
  - Acid may be added drop by drop
  - Add water till the volume becomes 1000 ml
  - Use it within 1 month
  - Useful only for hemoglobin estimation by the Sahli's method

Jaswant Singh and Bhattacharya (JSB) Stain

JSB Solution I

- Methylene blue   0.5 gm
- Sulfuric acid 1%   3.0 ml
- Potassium dichromate   0.5 gm
- Disodium hydrogen phosphate dihydrate   3.5 gm

- Distilled water   500 ml
  - Dissolve methylene blue in distilled water
  - Add sulfuric acid slowly, 1 ml at a time. Stirrer it constantly and mix well
  - Add potassium dichromate. There is formation of purple precipitate
  - Now add disodium hydrogen phosphate dehydrate. After stirring, it for some time precipitates get dissolved
  - Boil the solution in a flask with a reflux condensor for 1 hour when the blue color of solution deepens.

JSB Solution II

- Eosin (yellow, zinc free)   1.00 gm
- Distilled water   500 ml

Leishman Stain

- Leishman powder   1.5 gm
- Methanol   qs 1000 ml
  - Rinse out a clean bottle with methanol
  - Add a few clean dry glass beads
  - Add staining powder and then methanol
  - Mix well to dissolve the mixture
  - The stain thus prepared is kept as such and can be used next day
  - Take precautions, during preparation and storage of this strain, not to allow moisture to enter.

Lugol Iodine Solution

- Iodine   1 gm
- Potassium iodide   2 gm
- Distilled water   100 ml
  - Dissolve potassium iodide in about 30 ml of the water
  - Add iodine and mix until it is dissolved completely
  - Add 70 ml water and mix well
  - Store the solution in brown bottle.

Methylene Blue Aqueous

Solution for Ziehl-Neelsen Stain

- Methylene blue   0.5 gm

- Distilled water   100 ml
  - Mix methylene blue in 100 ml water
  - Filter after dissolving and store in bottle.

Ziehl-Neelsen Stain

- Methylene blue as prepared above   0.5 gm
- Borax   5.0 gm
- Distilled water   100 ml

Orthotolidine Reagent

- Orthotolidine dihydrochloride   1.35 gm
- Concentrated hydrochloric acid   150 ml
- Distilled water   850 ml
  - Distilled orthotolidine dihydrochloride in 500 ml of distilled water (Solution I)
  - Make a mixture of 350 ml of distilled water and 150 ml of concentrated hydrochloric acid (Solution II)
  - Add solution I and solution II with constant stirring
  - Store the solution in amber-colored bottles.

RBC Diluting Fluid

- Sodium citrate   3 gm
- Commercial formaldehyde solution   1 ml
  containing at least 37% formalin
- Distilled water   100 ml

Safranine Solution

Stock Solution

- Safranine O   2.5 gm
- Ethanol 95%   qs 100 ml

Working Solution

- Stock solution   10 ml
- Distilled water   900 ml

Sodium Chloride Solution (0.85%)

- Dissolve 0.85 gm sodium chloride in 1000 ml distilled water and store in bottle
- It is also called isotonic saline or normal saline.

Sodium Thiosulfate Aqueous Solution

- Sodium Thiosulfate anhydrous (for an equivalent quantity of $Na_2S_2O_3.5H_2O$) — 3 gm
- Distilled water — qs 100 ml
  - Mix and store in brown drop bottles
  - It is used to neutralize any chlorine in water samples taken for bacteriological analysis.

Sperm Diluting Fluid (Formalin-Bicarbonate)

- Sodium bicarbonate — 5 gm
- Commercial formaldehyde solution (formalin) — 1 gm
- Distilled water — 100 ml

WBC Diluting Fluid

- Acetic acid (CH_3COOH) glacial — 4 ml
- Distilled water — qs 200 ml
- Aqueous methylene blue solution — 10 drops
  - Dissolve 3.0 gm methylene blue in 100 ml of distilled water
  - Filter it
  - Add it to the acid solution (100 ml distilled water + 4 ml acetic acid).

Willis Solution

- Sodium chloride — 125 gm
- Distilled water — 500 ml
  - Dissolve sodium chloride by heating the mixture to boiling point
  - Leave to cool and wait
  - Some of the salt powder should remain undissolved
  - If all salt is dissolved, then add 50 gm sodium chloride more
  - Filter the solution and store in corked bottle
  - This is saturated solution of sodium chloride.

Drabkin's Solution

It is used for hemoglobin estimation. It contains:
- Potassium cyanide 500 mg
- Potassium ferricyanide 200 mg
- Potassium dehydrogen phosphate 140 mg
- Distilled water 1 liter
- pH 7.0-7.4

Indicator

Indicators in chemistry are compounds which are weak organic acids or bases. Depending upon the pH of the medium, these exist either in unionized form or ionized form. The two forms of the molecule have different colors. The color imparted to the medium by the indicators depend upon the relative proportions of unionized or ionized form of the indicator. The relative proportion of ionized or unionized form depends upon the pH of the medium and the dissociation constant (pK) of the indicator, as per the equation:

$$pH = pK + \log(salt/acid)$$

Since pK of an acid-base is constant, the ratio of salt to acid dependents on pH. The color of the undissociated and dissociated forms are different, so the color of the medium will be dependent on the ratio of the two forms, which is, in turn, dependent on pH.

To clarify we take the example of bromocresol green. The color of the undissociated form is yellow and that of dissociated is blue. The pK of bromocresol green is 4.7. At a pH of 4.7, the ratio of salt/acid is (i.e. both dissociated and undissociated forms are equal) and hence the equation:

$$pH = pK + \log(salt/acid)$$
$$pH = pK + \log 1 \ (\log 1 = 0)$$
$$pH = pK, \text{ i.e. } 4.7 = 4.7$$

Thus the color of the medium is green (i.e. equal amount of yellow and blue).

As the pH decreases, the yellow form of the indicator increases and at pH 3.8, it is almost pure yellow. Similarly, at pH 5.4, the indicator has pure blue color. In between pH 3.8 and 5.4, there exists a mixture of yellow or blue imparting various shades.

Selection of an indicator for determination of pH or during titration is usually on the basis of the range of pH likely to be encountered. For routine titration, the following indicators serve the purpose well.
- Strong acid versus strong base : Any indicator
- Strong acid versus weak base : Methyl orange
- Weak acid versus strong base : Phenolphthalein
- Weak acid versus weak base : No indicator is satisfactory

Preparation of Solutions in General

Percent Solution

To prepare a solution of a particular percentage, dissolve that much amount in grams in the required solvent, dilute it finally to 100 ml (W/V) or take the required volume in ml of the solute in liquid form, dissolve in the solvent and make the volume 100 ml with the solvent (V/V).

Note: Solvent is a medium in which a substance is dissolved, e.g. water.

Solute: The substance to be dissolved is called solute, e.g. when salt is dissolved in water, the salt is called the solute and water the solvent.

Solution: When solute is completely dissolved in a solvent, the resultant mixture is called solution.

Molar Solution

All compounds have their own molecular weight depending upon the number and proportion of component elements.

When molecular weight in grams of a substance is taken and dissolved in a solvent to a final volume of 1 liter, it makes molar solution accordingly twice the molecular weight in gram per liter will be two molar 2M, etc.

Normal Solution

Equivalent weight (molecular weight divided by valency) of a substance in grams dissolved per liter of solution is normal solution or 1 N. When the valency is one the molar solution is equal to normal solution, e.g. 40 gm of NaOH per liter of solution makes a molar or a normal solution. In case, the valency of an acid/base is two, the normal solution is half the molar solution, e.g. 74 gm of $Ca(OH)_2$ per liter makes a molar solution but 37 gm per liter are required to make a normal solution.

Preparation of Subnormal Solution

Solution of lower molarity or normality can be prepared from 1M/1N solution by the formula

$N_1V_1 = N_2V_2$
N_1 = Normality of solution I N_2 = Normality of solution II
V_1 = Volume of solution 1 V_2 = Final solution

Keep one side for the acid available and the other side for the solution finally to be made.

Molarity of sulfuric acid (H_2SO_4)

$$= \frac{W \times 1000}{T \times 381.4} = 2.62 \times \frac{W}{T}$$

Where, W = Weight of borax acid
T = Volume of acid used (ml)
381.4 = Molecular weight of borax acid

Now adjust the molarity according to the equation: $N_1V_1 = N_2V_2$

Examples

N/1 sulfuric acid is prepared as under:
Molecular weight of sulfuric acid = 2.016 + 64 + 32.066 = 98.082

$$\text{Equivalent weight} = \frac{\text{Molecular weight}}{2} = 49.041$$

- Therefore, N/1 sulfuric acid should contain 49.041 gm per liter
- Specific gravity is 1.84, therefore volume would be theoretically = 49.041/1.84
- Concentrated sulfuric acid contains only 95% pure acid and so volume of acid required is

$$\frac{49.041}{1.84} \times \frac{100}{95} = 28.1 \text{ ml}$$

Method

- Take 30 ml of concentrated sulfuric acid
- Pour slowly with stirring into 800 ml of water

- Cool and make upto 1000 ml
- Place 10 ml N/1 Na_2CO_3 (using volumetric pipette) in a beaker or flask
- Add a drop of methyl orange as an indicator
- Fill a burette with sulphuric acid and titrate the sodium bicarbonate with it until the color just changes to pink.

Calculation

- Suppose 9.5 ml of acid is required in the titration, then 9.5 ml acid is equivalent to $N/1.Na_2CO_3$
- To make a normal solution, add 0.5 ml water to each 9.5 ml of sulphuric acid

N/10 Sulfuric Acid

- Take 10 ml of N/1 sulfuric acid
- Dilute to 100 ml with distilled water.

N/1 Hydrochloric Acid

Molecular weight = H (1.008) + Cl (35.457) = 36.465

$$N/1 \text{ solution} = \frac{\text{Molecular weight}}{38 \times 1.18} = \frac{36.465}{0.4522} = 80.6 \text{ ml}$$

Specific gravity = 1.18, % of hydrochloric acid = 38, i.e. 80.6 ml of hydrochloric acid made up to 1000 ml to make N/1 hydrochloric acid.

Dilutions of Sample or Solution

Errors are usually made during calculations when samples or solutions are subjected to dilutions.

Double dilution: When one part or volume of a solution is mixed with one part or volume of diluent making a final volume of two (2 ml of blood + 2 ml saline = 4 ml).

Five times dilution: One part or volume of a sample or solution when mixed with four parts of diluent to make a final volume of five. Similarly, six times, seven times, ten times, etc.

Preparation of Standard Acids and Bases

Hydrochloric Acid (Approximately 1 mol/liter)

Titrate 90 ml of conc. HCl (sp. gr. 1.18) per liter. Titer it with sodium tetraborate ($Na_2B_4O_7 \cdot 10H_2O$, mol wt 381.4) using methyl red indicator and adjust accordingly.

Sulfuric Acid 1 M

Prepare an approximate 1 M solution of H_2SO_4 by taking 30 ml of concentrated acid. Add slowly to about 500 ml of water. Dilute finally to 1 liter and mix well. Standardize against borax and adjust accordingly.

Sodium Hydroxide 1 M

Quickly weight out 40 gm of solid sodium hydroxide and dissolve it in water and make it up to 1 liter. This makes an approximate 1 M solution. Titrate it with standardized in HCl or the H_2SO_4 using phenolphthalein as an indicator.

Standardization Against Borax

Weight out accurately about 4 mg of borax (Sodium tetraborate, $Na_2B_4O_7 \cdot 10H_2O$). Transfer it to a conical flask and dissolve it by warming in about 100 ml water. Add a few drops of methyl red indicator and titrate it with HCl or H_2SO_4 to find out the molarity of the acid, using the following equation:

$$\text{Molarity of HCl} = \frac{2W \times 1000}{T \times 381.4} = 5.24 \times \frac{W}{T}$$

$$= \frac{W \times 1000}{T \times 381.7}$$

SI Units

To have uniformity in expression of analytical results in clinical chemistry, a system was adopted in 1966 based on SI units (System International d'Units) by International Federation of Clinical Chemistry and approved in 1967. The seven basic SI units are as follows:

Section 1: Medical Laboratory

Quantity	Unit	Symbol
Length	Meter	M
Mass	Kilogram	kg
Time	Second	sec
Current	Ampere	A
Thermodynamic temperature	Kelvin	K
Amount of substance	Mole	Mol
Luminous intensity	Candela	cd

These are recommended prefixes used to form decimal multiples and submultiples of SI units, such as deca (da) =10^1, hectare (h) =10^2, kilo (K) =10^3 or milli (m) =10^{-3}, micro (µ) =10^{-6}, nano =(n) =10^{-9}, etc.

The decimal sign between digits is indicated by a full stop. A zero should recede the decimal sign if numerical sign is less than 1. The use of such expressions as 0.003 mol/L is not recommended rather it should be expressed as 3 mmol/L.

CHAPTER 2

Laboratory Equipment

Microscope

Human eye can see an object upto 30 mm only. Undoubtedly, microscope is one of the most important equipment in the hospital laboratory. It makes small objects appear larger than they actually are, so that details of the objects can be seen, which otherwise is not possible. It does so by the use of lenses like the ordinary magnifying glass.

Construction

The laboratory microscope has three main parts: Microscope stand, mechanical adjustments and the optics or lenses (**Fig. 2.1**).

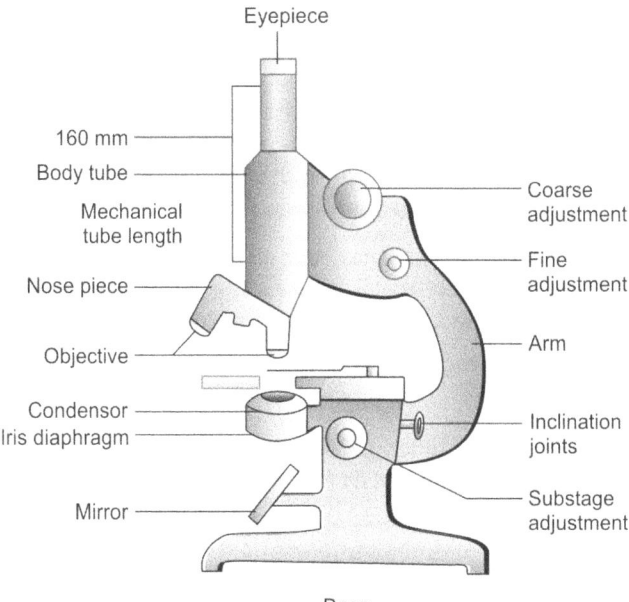

Fig. 2.1: Microscope

The microscope stand: It provides metal support for all other parts of microscope. It consists of: (i) the tube which holds the objectives and the eyepiece; (ii) the body which is concerned with their focusing; (iii) the arm which support all these; (iv) the stage on which specimen lies; and (v) the foot or base on which the whole instrument rests. These are discussed as under:

The tube: It supports at its lower end the objective and at its upper end the eyepiece. It holds these in line and the correct distance apart. The objective is screwed into the lower end of the tube. Usually, for laboratory work about 30 objectives are screwed into revolving nose piece, which allows any of the objectives to be quickly adjusted into place. The eyepiece is inserted loosely into the upper end of the tube. Eyepiece also has standard diameter so that eyepieces are interchangeable. Also eyepieces are moveable up or down in a sliding draw tube at the upper end of the tube.

The body: The tube is attached to the microscope by the body. The body is a block of metal containing the focussing mechanism.

The arm: The body of the microscope and the tube attached to it are supported at the correct height and tilted to required angle by firm arm which usually provides a lifting handle for the microscope.

The stage: This is a flat plate lying below the objective, on which specimen or object to be examined, is placed. It carries a pair of spring stage clips which hold it in place. In the center of the stage, there is a circular hole for the light to pass upward through it from below.

Mechanical stage: The stage may have attached to its upper surface of may incorporate a mechanical stage for the controlled movement of the specimen. In this case, stage clips are absent.

The substage: It lies just below the stage. It holds a condenser lens, iris diaphragm and holder for light filters and stops.

The foot: It may be of different forms, i.e. horseshoe, tripod, etc. As a matter of fact, microscope rests firmly on a foot upon the laboratory bench.

Mechanical Adjustments

It includes focussing of the objectives, adjustment of the mirror, condenser, iris and also the use of the drawtube and other movements.

Focusing adjustment: The quality of operation of microscope depends also on the perfect movement of its focusing mechanisms (coarse, fine). These focusing adjustments operate by a strip of metal sliding up and down in a matching slot carefully machined and lubricated to give smooth and easy movements.

The coarse adjustment is driven by a rack and pinion mechanism. It is generally controlled by a pair of large knobs, lying one on each side of the body. By rotating it, the tube with lenses moves. In some microscopes, the stage moves up and down rapidly. As a matter of fact, coarse adjustment is the focusing of low power lenses.

The fine adjustment is brought about by a micrometer thread. Here, high power lens requires fine adjustment, the knobs move the objectives or the stage up or down extremely slow. The two smaller knobs on each side of the body, may be graduates in micron to show the distance moved.

The Microscope Optics

Objectives

The objective is most important part of microscope. Usually, there are three objectives (**Fig. 2.2**):
1. 10X   (low power)
2. 45X   (high power)
3. 100X (oil immersion)

Eyepiece

The most common form of eyepiece is Huyghens' eyepiece. Huyghens' eyepieces are available in a range of magnifications 4X, 6X, 7X, 8X, 10X, 15X and sometimes 20X. The higher, the power, the greater is the total magnification of microscope. The lower the power of eyepiece, the brighter and sharper is the image. 10X eyepiece is a good average lens, giving sufficient magnification and details for routine work (**Fig. 2.3**).

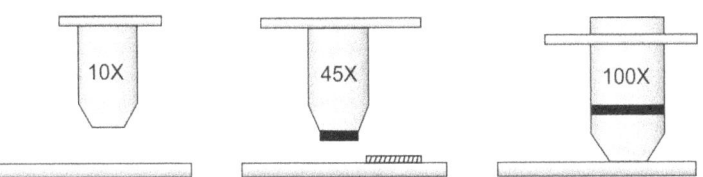

Fig. 2.2: Objectives

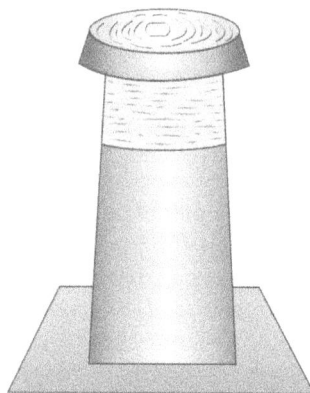

Fig. 2.3: Eyepiece

Condenser and Iris

The condenser is a large lens mounted below the stage with an iris diaphragm. This lens receives a beam from light and passes it into the objective. The angle of beam can be adjusted by iris (**Fig. 2.4**).

Mirror

Below condenser and iris is the mirror which is circular and mounted so that it can be turned in any direction and will stay in place. It reflects the light from source of light (sunlight, electric light, etc.) upwards through the iris into the condenser. It consists of two mirrors, mounted back to

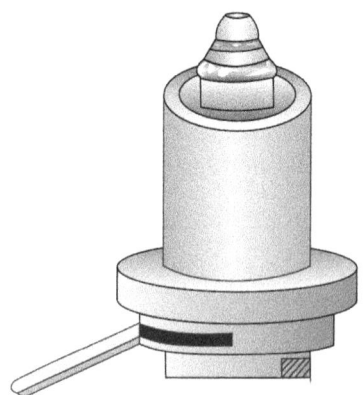

Fig. 2.4: Condenser

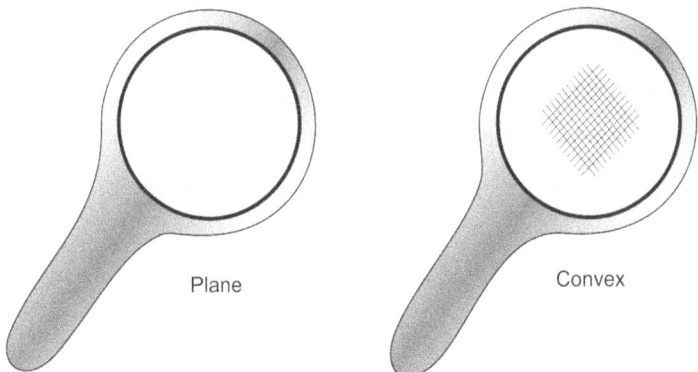

Fig. 2.5: Mirror

back. One of these, two mirrors is plane or flat and the other is concave. The flat mirror is used with condenser whereas plane mirror is used without condenser (**Fig. 2.5**).

Drawtube

The tube length is adjusted simply by sliding the drawtube with its eyepiece up or down. The drawtube is usually 160 mm. Objectives work best at this tube length.

Inclination

The arm can be tilted upon the foot by hinge, which may have a clamping screw, to allow the tube and the stage to be inclined together to an angle as required.

Condenser Adjustment

The condenser has necessary adjustments for its focusing, for its aperture and for its centering too. It can also be swing aside (for removal or to exchange it by a new one). Just below condenser is a holder for variety of filters.

The condenser is usually moved up and down for focusing by rotating a knob to one side of it and below the stage.

Aperture Adjustment

The aperture is adjusted by the iris diaphragm which lies just below the condenser. It can be closed or opened as required, by moving a small projecting knob.

Mechanical Stage

It holds the slide in place and moves it smoothly in a straight line either across or along the stage with knobs, one for each direction. There is also measuring scale for each movement.

Source of Light

It may be natural sunlight or artificial light, i.e. electric bulb (**Fig. 2.6**). Electric bulb should be of 60 watt placed 18 inches away from microscope.

Routine Use of Microscope

- Place the microscope on firm bench so that it does not vibrate
- If source of light is sun, flat side of mirror is used to reflect the light up through the condenser
- Place the specimen on the stage and examine under low power (10X) and then under high power (45X). Specimen to be examined under oil immersion lens (100X) should be examined after placing a drop of cedarwood oil

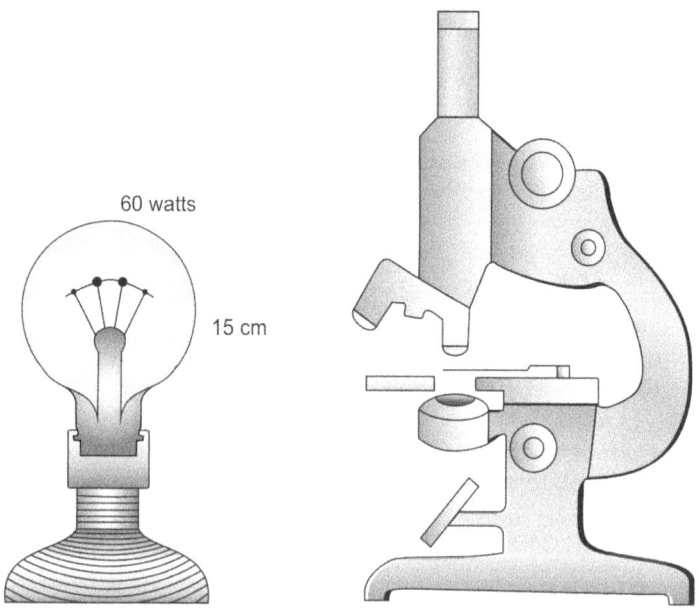

Fig. 2.6: Light source

- Focus the objective using coarse focusing knob until the lens (objective) is near the specimen. Now use the fine focusing knob until sharp image comes into view
- Turn the mirror until the illumination of image is at its brightest
- Adjust and condenser, aperture of condenser and iris. Usually for stained specimen on slide, wide aperture is used. Reduced aperture is used to increase the contrast for usually unstained preparation on slide mounted in saline and under a coverslip
- Now examine the slide moving it by mechanical stage.

Phase Contrast Microscopy (Figs. 2.7 and 2.8)

- The structures within cells have different thickness that inturn gives good contrast.
- The difference in thickness between bacterial cell and surrounding medium makes them clearly visible. Reduction by fraction of the wavelength of rays of light that pass through the bacterial cell is compared to the rays that is passing through the surrounding medium which produces a phase difference between the two types of rays. In short, these phase differences are converted into differences in intensity of light.
- This produces light and dark contrast image.
- With this type of microscope, we can study structures within cell.
- Phase contrast microscope has the advantage of studying living organisms.

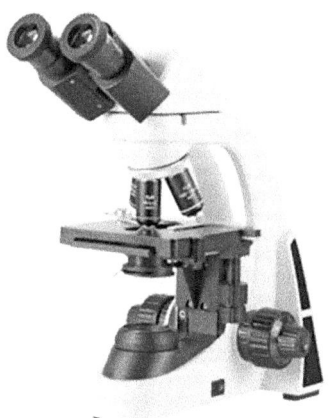

Fig. 2.7: Compound binocular microscope

Section 1: Medical Laboratory

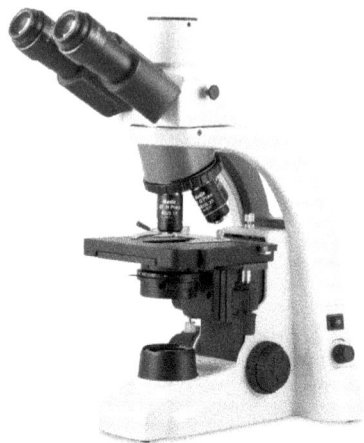

Fig. 2.8: Phase contrast microscope

- Phase contrast microscope has specific application in the identification of fungi.

Dark Ground Microscope (Fig. 2.9)
- Bacteria can be seen in living state.
- As we use reflected light we get better contrast. It is not possible if we use transmitted light.

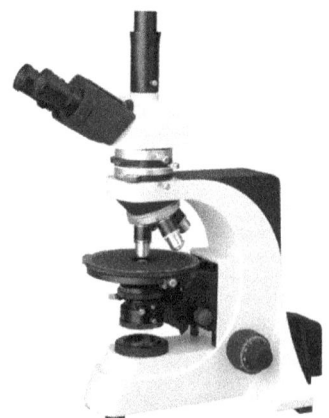

Fig. 2.9: Dark ground microscope

Chapter 2: Laboratory Equipment

- Dark field condenser is a special part of this microscope. It has central circular stop. It illuminates the object with the cone of light. It does not allow any ray of light fall directly on the object.
- Rays of light falling on the object are scattered on the objective lens, making object self-luminous against dark background. Thus, we get illusion of increased resolution. Hence, we can see very thin organisms like *Treponema pallidum*.

Polarizing Microscope (Fig. 2.10)

- In polarizing microscope two prisms are used, one below the condenser and other above the objective.

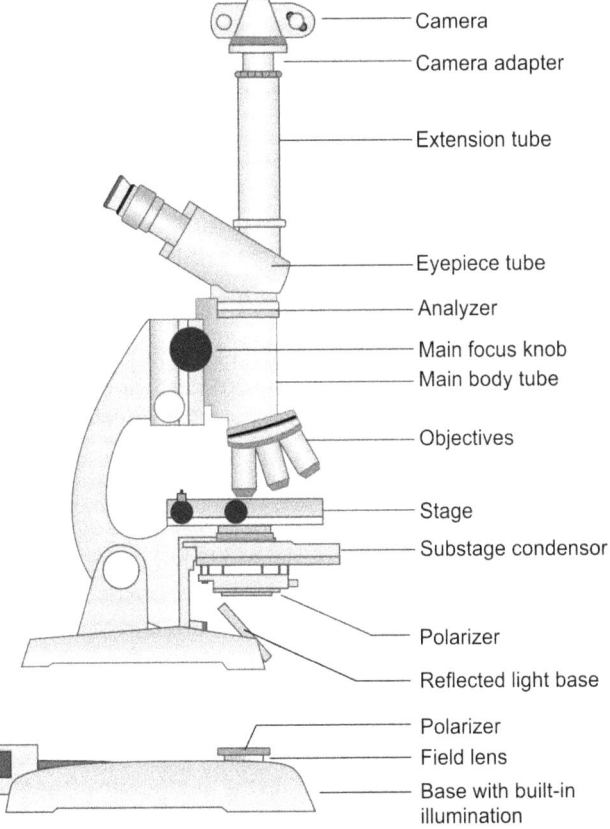

Fig. 2.10: Polarizing microscope

- When both are crossed, no light passes through the upper prism.
- If cholesterol crystals are placed at the object plane, the light rays that pass through these crystals can pass through the upper prism. It is because the prisms are not crossed for these rays
- The rays that fail to pass through these crystals are absorbed by upper prism. Thus, these cholesterol crystals are seen as bright objects against background.
- Polarizing microscope works on the principle that upward and downward vibration of particles results in producing wave motion. These particles move in any direction at right angle to the direction of light. On passing light ray through Nicol's prism, it becomes polarized and it moves in one direction only. The ray through another prism in the path will pass unchanged. It happens only if the optical path of second prism is in alignment with the former. In case, second prism is rotated through 90°, such that their optical path are crossed then the ray will be totally reflected out of second prism. Hence no light will pass through crossed prisms.
- Polarizing microscope may be used to demonstrate birefringent objects like cholesterol crystals, amyloid teeth, striated bone, muscle tissue, neurons, etc.

Electron Microscope (Fig. 2.11)

In this microscope, electrons are used as a source of light. Since wavelength of electrons is very small (0.005 nm), the resolution power of electron microscope is greatly increased. The wavelength of visible light is 500 nm.

Construction

- Electromagnet are analogous to lens of light microscope.
- It consists of electromagnetic fields whose power can be changed.
- The object under examination must be ultra-thin as electrons have poor penetration power.
- Electrons generated at the top of cathode tube gets converted by an electromagnetic field (condenser) on to the object.
- The objective of electron microscope field produces an enlarged image of the object which falls within the focal length of the eyepiece.
- The latter magnifies the image larger, and the image is either photographed or seen by using fluorescent screen.

Chapter 2: Laboratory Equipment

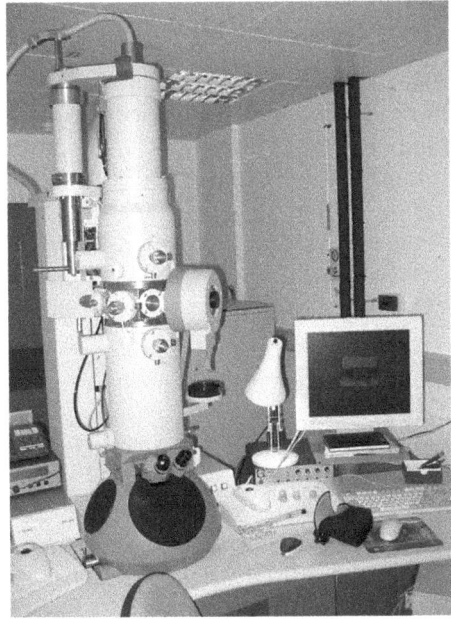

Fig. 2.11: Electron microscope

- Those parts of tissue that are electron dense allow less number of electrons to pass through and hence less change in graphic plate.
- When the positive print of photographic plate is made, electron denser objects appear as dark bodies and those objects with few number of electrons look lighter.

Uses

- Since electron microscope has extremely great resolution power (0.1 nm), ultramicroscope objects are observed and studied with ease, e.g. viruses.
- This microscope makes it possible to study cellular structure. Hence, it is very useful for research purposes.

Interference Microscope

- We can study the organelles.
- Further we can collect information regarding quantitative measurements of chemicals of cell like lipid, proteomics and nucleic acids.

Photometer or Colorimeter

Though in routine, the name colorimeter is given to the equipment used to measure optical density or absorbance of colored solution but actually these should be named as photometers or spectrophotometers. Photometers are either single cell or double cell depending upon one or two photo devices in the photometers. Depending upon the arrangement of obtaining monochromatic light, the photometers are called as filter-photometers or spectrophotometers. Since, single cell filter photometers are common in use a general structure of the one is described.

Construction

The colorimeter or photometer has basically six components (**Figs 2.12 and 2.13**):
1. Light source is a low wattage 6–12 volt ordinary bulb operated on a battery or through step-down transformer. A reflector (concave mirror) reflects a parallel beam of light which finally passes through the sample.

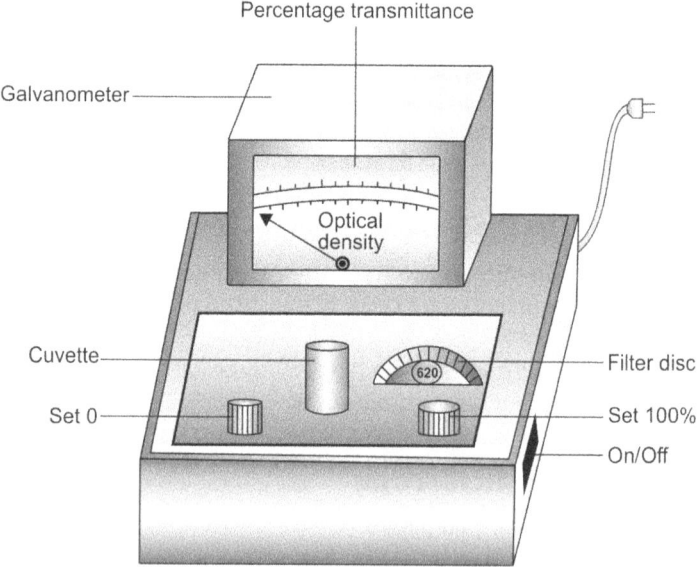

Fig. 2.12: Single cell filter photometer (schematic)

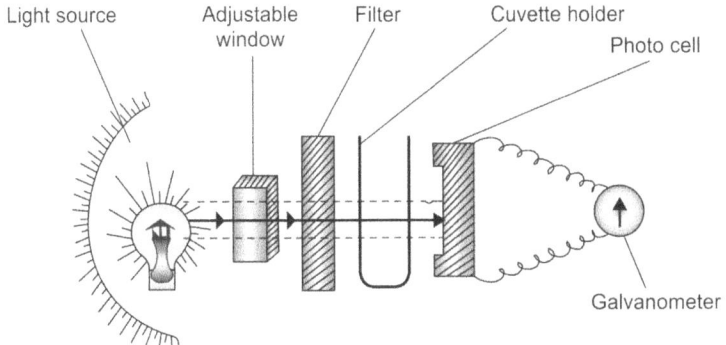

Fig. 2.13: Schematic diagram of a single cell filter photo cell

2. Light adjustment is done by passing the beam of light through an adjustable window or diaphragm where aperture can be adjusted to make less or more light to pass through.
3. Wavelength selection is made by filters which are either mounted on a circular disc which can be rotated to bring the required filter in the path of light or the required filters can be inserted directly in the path of light.
4. The sample whose absorbance is to be measured is taken in a cuvette, which is put in a cuvette holder. The cuvette holder has two slits for the passage of light beam, one at the incident and other at the emergent surface. The cuvettes are either cylindrical or rectangular.
5. The conversion of light energy into electrical energy is accomplished by a photoelectric cell or "photocell" or in more sophisticated instruments by photoemissive tubes.
6. Light falling on the photocell is converted into electrical current, which is measured by a galvanometer.

The galvanometer needle moves over a scale which is equally divided from 0-100 division and corresponds to % transmittance. Another scale superimposed on this scale is that of 'optical density' or absorbance which is related to % transmittance as $2-\log G$. Some photometers have galvanometers which give direct digital display giving the reading as % transmittance or optical density.

Operation of Photometers

- Connect the photometer to the mains preferably through a constant voltage stabilizer
- Switch on the instrument

Section 1: Medical Laboratory

- Move the filter wheel to bring the desired filter in position or place the required filter in the filter place
- Fill the cuvette with reagent blank or water and place it in the cuvette holder
- Adjust the light intensity to set the pointer 100% transmittance or zero optical density
- Remove the cuvette. Fill standard or sample, colored solution in place of water (or blank). Replace the cuvette in the cuvette holder. The needle will move towards the left on the scale
- Read absorbance or optical density from the scale directly
- Read the absorbance of the other samples
- Check zero after taking a few reading
- Switch off the instrument as soon as the readings are over.

Autoclave

Construction

It has a vertical gunmetal chamber with strong gunmetal lid. This lid lies over the chamber and can be air-tightened with screw nuts or rubber gasket. An air and steam discharge tap, pressure gauge and safety valve are fitted with the lid. The chamber carries heater coil at its bottom (**Fig. 2.14**).

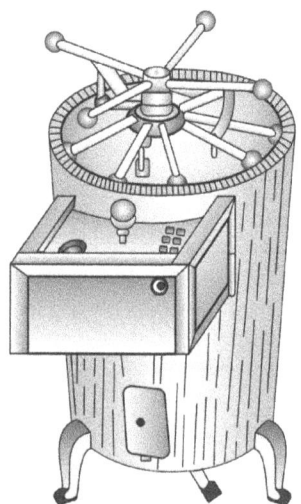

Fig. 2.14: Vertical autoclave

Operation of Autoclave

- Keep the required amount of water at the bottom of the chamber
- Keep the articles to be sterilized inside the autoclave. On perforated plate lying above the level of water
- Close the lid of autoclave tightly and switch on the autoclave
- Keep the air-cum-steam discharge tap open till steam starts coming through it
- Close air-cum-steam discharge tap
- Now, wait till pressure gauze shows 20 lbs per square inch pressure.
- Wait for 20 minutes
- Now switch off autoclave and slowly open steam discharge tap
- Let the steam come out for some time
- When pressure gauze shows zero reading, open the lid and bring out the sterilized material.

Biological Safety Cabinet

It protects the laboratory worker from the harmful effects while working with infectious or chemical material. It also protects experimental material from getting contaminated. As a matter of fact, this equipment is ideal for working with infectious material, e.g. aspirating infectious material with syringe, etc. This safety cabinet may also be used when working with human blood, body fluids, and maintaining sterile cells and tissue culture.

The biological safety cabinet is enclosed box. It is leak-free box with gloves. It uses vertical laminar airflow having a barrier of protection against airborne micro-organisms in the form of high efficiency particulate air (HEPA). This filter removes airborne particles including micro-organisms going into working area and out to environment. Thus, it creates sterile work environment.

Types of Safety Cabinets

Mainly, there are following three types of biological safety cabinets:

Class I

They have open front air inflow. They provide good protection for worker. However, there is no product protection. Here, filtered air is not provided over working area.

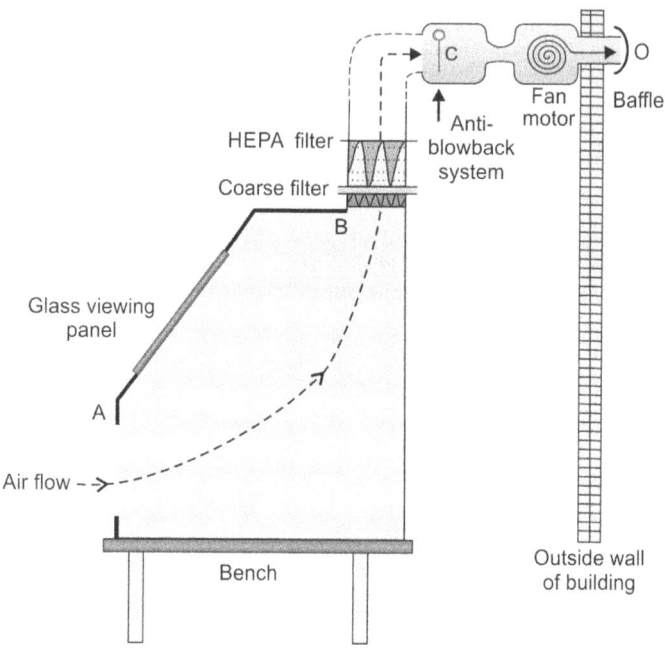

Fig. 2.15: A class 1 microbiological safety cabinet. Air is drawn through the cabinet (A) through a HEPA filter in the exhaust trunking at (B), and then via an anti-blowback system at (C) to be discharged at (D). The exhaust fan must be close to the discharging point.

Air enters the cabinet through (A) and passes through HEPA filter exhaust trunking at (B). Now air enters anti-blowback system at (C) to be discharged at (D) (**Fig. 2.15**).

Class 2

They provide protection both for the worker and working area. A downward flow of air flushes working area and directs the air an inward flow at the front opening (A). The air may be totally recirculated or totally exhausted. There are four subtypes of class 2 cabinet based on construction, inflow air velocities and exhaust system (**Fig. 2.16**).

Class 3

They are totally enclosed, airtight ventilated cabinets. The work operation conducted through fixed attached rubber gloves (**Fig. 2.17**).

Chapter 2: Laboratory Equipment

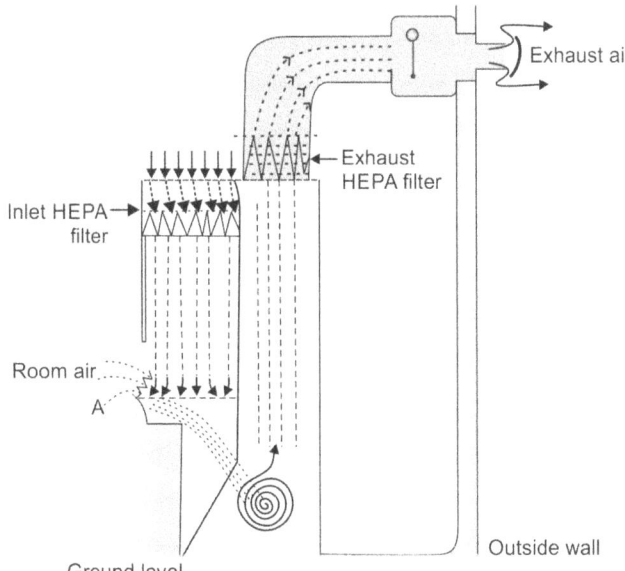

Fig. 2.16: A unidirectional downward flow of filtered air flushes the working area and induces an inward flow at the front opening (A). The air may be partially recirculated it may be totally exhausted as shown have in simplified outline.

Operation Procedure

- Put on cabinet blower for 5 minutes to remove particulates from the cabinet
- Wipe and clean carefully the work surface, interior wall and surface of the window
- Place only the items inside cabinet which are actually required during procedure
- Use protective clothing, e.g. laboratory coat while working with cabinet
- Avoid making rapid movements of arms while working
- Instead of open flame use touch plate burner
- Preferably sterile tools should be used while working in the cabinet
- When work is finished, all the items within the cabinet should be wiped carefully and properly with disinfectant. After this, they must be removed from cabinet
- Check the HEPA filter periodically

Section 1: Medical Laboratory

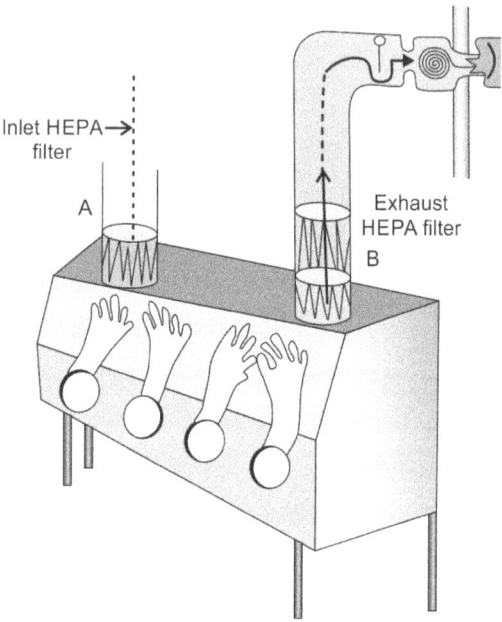

Fig. 2.17: Safety cabinet with A-glove ports filtered air is continuously drawn into the totally enclosed cabinet via a HEPA filter (A) and exhausted through HEPA filters (B). The gloves are fixed to the ports so the operations are separated from the work. Materials and equipment to be handled within the cabinet are admitted via ports that air then sealed by doors closing on to airtight gaskets

- Put on ultraviolet light 45 minutes before starting the work in the cabinet
- Make it a must to put off ultraviolet light before actually working. As a matter of fact, ultraviolet rays may damage the retina and skin.

Laminar Airflow

Here horizontal laminar airflow clean benches. As a matter of fact, it discharges HEPA filtered air across the work surface and toward the worker. Hence, this equipment provides only product protection. Its utility can be made to create clean working conditions, e.g. dust-free assembly of sterile equipment or electronic material (**Fig. 2.18**).

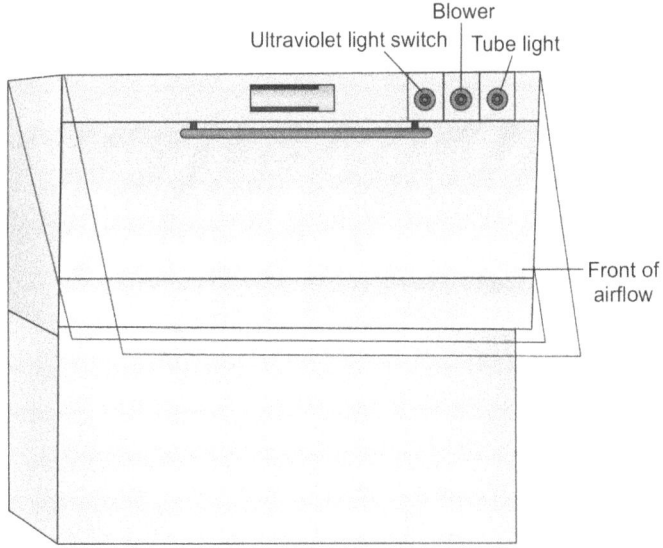

Fig. 2.18: Laminar airflow (Clean benches)

Differences between Laminar Airflow and Biological Safety Cabinet

Laminar airflow	Biological safety cabinet
It is clean benches	It provides personnel environment and product protection
It discharges HEPA-filtered air across work area and towards user	HEPA filter is used in exhaust and or supply system to filter the air in the biological safety cabinet
It reduces turbulence area and minimizes the potential for cross-contamination	It completely protects form airborne contamination
It has no leak-free boxes and gloves	It may have leak-free boxes with gloves sealing the hand holes

Hot Air Oven

Construction

It is double-layered chamber. It is divided into three compartments by two perforated plates. Its bottom carries coils of heater. It carries on/off switch and thermostat control. It has a door (**Fig. 2.19**).

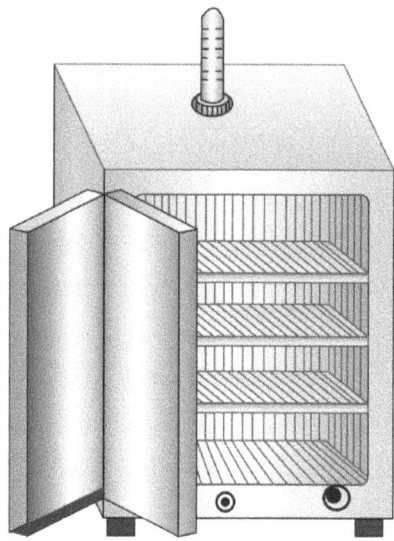

Fig. 2.19: Hot air oven

Operation of Hot Air Oven

- Put the articles to be sterilized after properly drying and packing them inside the chamber
- Close the door and adjust the temperature required with the help of thermostat
- Switch on the apparatus and wait till the required temperature is attained (160°C)
- Wait for 1 hour and after it switch off the apparatus
- Wait till temperature comes down to room temperature
- Take out the articles and use them according to requirement.
  Other methods of sterilization are filtration, radiations, chemicals, etc.

Centrifuge Machine

Centrifuge is used to deposit rapidly particles, such as cells which are suspended in a fluid. It can be done by spinning the tubes of fluid in centrifuge bucket using centrifugal force. The speed is expressed as the number of revolutions per minute (**Fig. 2.20**).

Principle: This equipment works on the principle of centrifugal force.

Chapter 2: Laboratory Equipment

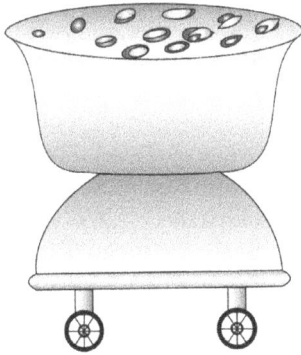

Fig. 2.20: Centrifuge machine

Construction

The centrifuge machine consists of a central vertical pillar. From this pillar, number of arms extend diametrically across. At the end of each arm is suspended a conical metal bucket. All buckets are of same size, weight and they are exactly at equal distance from the vertical pillar. Each bucket holds centrifuge tube. These tubes are also of same size and weight. The centrifuge tubes placed opposite each others in the centrifuge must contain equal amount of fluid. The centrifuge machine can be moved at various revolutions per minute, usually 3000 revolutions per minute (**Fig. 2.15**).

How to Use Centrifuge?

- Apparatus must be placed on a firm base
- The cups or buckets must be balanced in pairs
- Test tubes should be matched against one another in respect of size, weight, thickness of glass, contents, etc.
- Centers of gravity of tubes must be at equal radial distances
- Final adjustment of balance of tubes and bucket should be made on a rough balance by adding a few drops of water to the buckets. If balance of tubes and bucket is not maintained, motor of centrifuge may get damaged
- Centrifuge bowl should be kept clean and if a tube is accidentally broken, one should make it sure to clean the centrifuge before using it again
- The centrifuge machine should be operated with its cover or lid in place, otherwise it will reduce its speed

- Cotton-wool should never be used as a stopper for tubes during centrifugation
- Centrifuge must be started slowly and then the speed is increased.

Precautions

- As discussed, tubes in centrifuge must be balanced properly. If it is not done so, tubes get broken
- Do not increase or decrease the speed of the centrifuge too rapidly
- Do not touch the centrifuge when it is in operation.

Other Types of Centrifuge Machine

Hand Centrifuge

It can be operated with handle which can be moved with hand at a speed upto 2000 to 2500 revolutions per minute. It has 2 to 4 buckets, which are made up of aluminium each with the capacity of 15 ml.

Electric Centrifuge

These machines are available in horizontal swing out head. They can reach upto 3000 revolutions per minute with built in multistage speed regulator to obtain desired speed.

Balance

A balance is used to find the mass of a body by comparing it with known mass. A spring balance measures the weight of the body, by distortion of the spring.

Rough Balance

It is used for weighing out substances where great accuracy is not required. It usually is an open balance which may have one pan or two pans. It usually weighs to the nearest 100 mg.

Analytic Balance

It is highly sensitive and delicate instrument. It can weigh to the nearest 1 mg or less. The balance is enclosed in a case at all times and the doors (sliding doors) should be closed while weighing so that small air currents do not move pans and cause errors. This balance is used where utmost accuracy is required. It is usually used for weighing material required for the preparation of reagents, etc.

Construction of Analytic Balance

Analytic balance consists of a beam supported at the center by a knife-edge made up of steel or agate. This knife-edge rests on a plate of hard material fixed to the top of a support which moves inside the pillar. At the two ends of the beam and at equal distances from the central knife-edge, there are two knife-edges pointing upwards. From these are hung two stirrups which carry scale pans of equal masses. A pointer is attached to the middle of the beam perpendicular to it and this moves over an ivory scale fixed at the bottom of the pillar. The beam is kept in an arrested position when balance is not used. The beam can be arrested or released by turning a handle. There are two adjusting nuts at the ends, by adjusting which the pointer can be made to swing within the scale. The balance is mounted on a wooden platform provided with two leveling screws so as to make the pillar vertical and this is indicated by the plummet (**Fig. 2.21**).

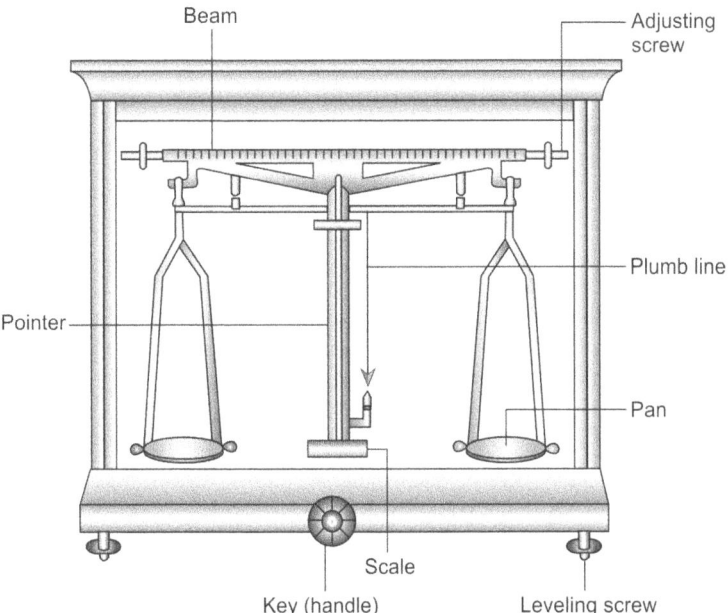

Fig. 2.21: Analytic balance

Sensitivity of a balance is defined as the shift in the resting point of the balance due to the addition of a small load (usually 1 mg). The weight box supplied with an analytic balance ordinarily consists of the following standard masses or weights:

100 gm	50 gm	20 gm	10 gm	5 gm	2 gm
1 gm	500 mg	200 mg	100 mg	50 mg	20 mg
10 mg					

The weight box contains a pair of forceps. The weights are always to be taken with the forceps and never with the hand. Keep the weight in the right pan and chemicals to be weighed on the left pan.

Working of Balance

- Adjust the leveling screws till the plummet comes exactly over the index, so that the pillar may become vertical
- Using soft brush remove dust from pans
- Release the beam by gently turning the handle. Beam must be resting on its knife edge. Make the pointer to move within the ivory scale by carefully adjusting the screw nuts at the ends of the beam
- The object to be weighed should be placed in the left pan and standard masses from weight box in the right pan
- The weights should be added in descending order of magnitude (heavy weight first followed by less weight)
- The beam of the balance should be arrested when not in use and also before adding or removing weights
- The balance should be arrested gently without any jerks
- The weights should not be left to lie about but should remain in the scale pan only when required. Alternatively, they should be kept in weight box
- The standard weight should not be touched with the hands, but only with the forceps
- The balance should not be loaded with weight greater than the maximum it is constructed to weigh
- The object should not be weighed hot
- Whenever a reading is taken, the balance case should be kept closed.

Care of Balance

- Balance should be kept in a glasses case. Thus, moisture of air cannot damage it. Dust can also not settle on it
- If any substance is spilled on a scale pan, the pan should be removed and thoroughly cleaned

- Balance should be cleaned with small hair brush
- Nothing should be placed on, or removed from either scale pans, while the scale pans are swinging. Beam of the balance should be arrested when the balance is not in use and also before adding or removing weight
- Balance is not jerked in any manner. The scale pans should be raised and lowered by arresting the beam gently and only when the pointer is nearly at its equilibrium state
- Every care should be taken to avoid powder sticking to the bottom of scale pan
- The balance should not be loaded with a weight greater than the maximum, it is constructed for. Use of more than the maximum weight allowed, may damage the sensitivity of balance
- Weights should not be toughed with the fingers, but should be lifted with the forceps provided with each box of weights. Otherwise moisture, grease, or other dirt from finger may cling to weight. Thus, affecting the accuracy, i.e. 1 gm weight may actually become 1.1 gm. For cleaning pans, silk piece should be used as ordinary duster may leave threads of cotton.

Autoanalyzer

The analyzer is fully automated. The analyzer is discrete, computerized. It uses serum/plasma, urine, CSF, and supernatant samples. Auto- analyzer performs in vitro quantitative and qualitative test on wide range (**Fig. 2.22**).

Analyzer is composed of two hardware units as under:
1. The analytical unit
2. Control unit

The Analytical Unit

- The ISE system
- Photometric measuring system
- The analytical processing unit (**Fig. 2.23**)

Control Unit

- Color monitor with touch screen
- Keyboard and trach ball
- Printer
- Central processing unit (CPU)

Section 1: Medical Laboratory

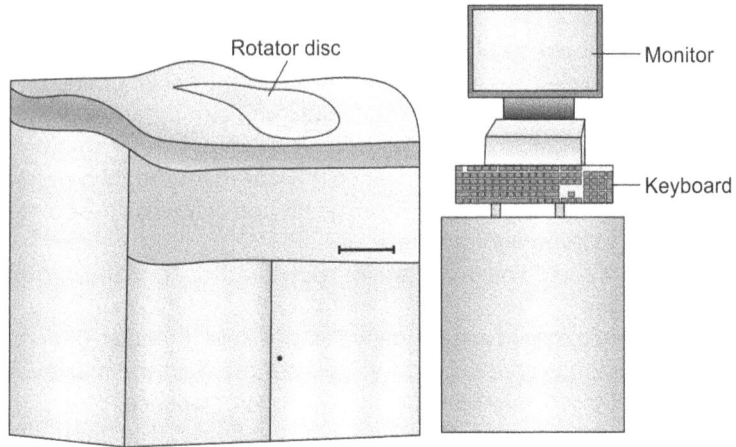

Fig. 2.22: Autoanalyzer

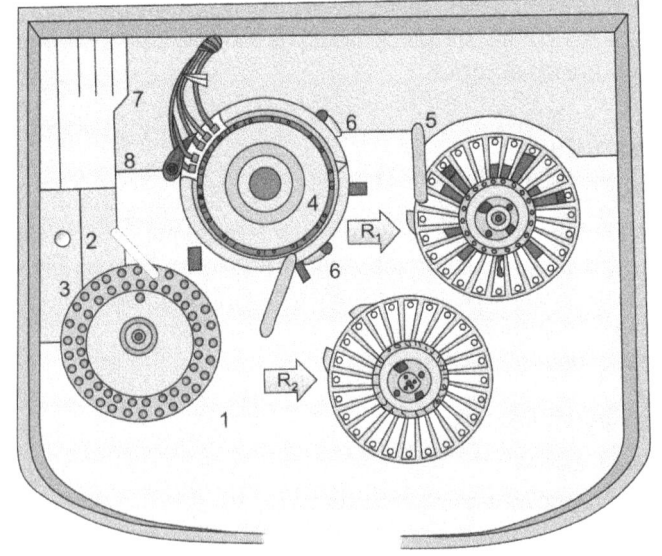

1. Sample disc
2. Sample probe
3. ISE dilution vessel
4. Reaction disk/incubation bath
5. Reagent probes
6. Stirring paddles
7. Photometer
8. Cell rinse unit

Fig. 2.23: The analytical unit

Characteristics

Analyzer characteristics include:
- Ready to use 24 hours
- Sample bar code capability
- Reagent bar code capability
- 360 tests/hour throughput
- Automatic calibration performance followed by quantity control
- Automatic sample blanking
- Automatic sample dilution capabilities
- Refrigerated storage for 64 reagent containers
- 115 position for routine, stat calibrator and quantity control sample and wash solution
- Automatic rerun capability.

Analyzer Operational Systems

The analyzer uses several operational systems. These systems include:
- Control system
- Sampling system
- Reagent system
- Photometric measuring system
- Cell rinse system

Procedure

- The sample disc rotates the appropriate sample to the sample probe
- The sample probe aspirates sample for testing
- After the sample is placed into the reaction cell, reagent probes add up to four different reagents separate dispense cycles
- Stirring paddles mix the sample after the addition of each reagent
- Incubation occurs as cells are immersed in the incubation both below the reaction disc. Cells rotate the photometer light path and a measurement taken
- The cell rinse unit removes product waste and washes, rinse and blanks cells.

Advantages

- Readily available for use
- Capability of processing over 720 tests per hour
- Automatic calibrations performance

- 115 positions for routine, stat calibrator, blood samples and wash solution
- Automatic return capability.

Disadvantages

- Not suitable for small number of samples
- Require proper training of staff about working maintenance and potential problems of machine
- Equipment is expensive and so is its maintenance.

Precautions

- Washing of analyzer daily
- Do not touch the solution during processing
- Do not switch off the equipment directly
- Do not put the sample in the equipment during it working

Inspissator

Principle

Inspissator works on the principle of wet heating at temperature below 100°C (**Fig. 2.24**).

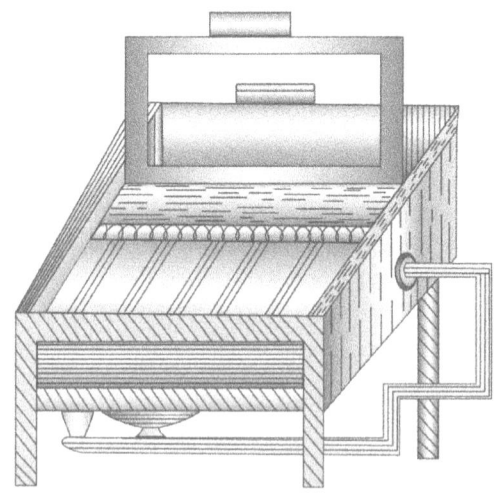

Fig. 2.24: Inspissator

Construction

- Inspissator consists of a double wall copper box
- Water flows between two walls
- Thermostat is also fitted within two walls
- Inside, it has sloping racks to hold tubes in slanting position
- It has lid made up a clear glass
- Base is fitted with heating coils to heat it.

Operation

- Keep the media containing tubes in sloping racks
- Close the glass lid
- Put on electric switch
- Fix the temperature between 75°C and 85°C
- Media containing tubes are maintained at this temperature for 1 hour daily for 3 days
- To prevent drying of medium, holes are provided in the chamber at a level higher than that of water. Thus, water vapors keep the medium moist.

Precautions

- Check the water levels of inspissator before putting it on
- Keep media containing bottle properly on sloping rack
- Put on the switch after closing the lid or door of inspissator
- Note down the temperature when it reaches 75 to 80°C and then wait for 2 to 3 hours
- Put off the switch and then put on switch next day. Repeat it for 3 days
- Do not touch or open inspissator when inspissator is on.

Uses

- Used to sterilize media containing serum, e.g. Loeffler serum slope
- Media containing egg can also be sterilized, e.g. Löwenstein-Jensen egg medium
- Media can be prepared in the form of slope.

Wood's Lamp (Fig. 2.25)

- It was invented in 1903 by Robert W Wood (physicist)

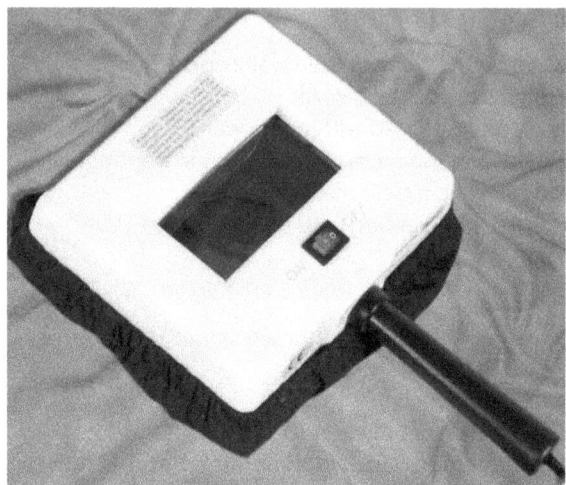

Fig. 2.25: Wood's lamp

- It is used mainly for the detection of fungal infection. First used by Margarot and Deveze in 1925 for the detection of fungal infection of hour.

Wood's lamp is small durable, inexpensive, safe and easy to use. It emits long wave ultraviolet radiation (also named black light), generated by high pressure mercury arc fitted with a compound filter made up of barium silicate with 9% nickel oxide. This filter is opaque to all light rays except a band between 320 and 400 nm with a peak at 365 nm. Fluorescence of tissue occurs when wood's light is absorbed and radiation of a longer wavelength, usually visible light is emitted. The output of Wood's lamp is usually low (<1 m ω/cm^2)

Technique of Wood's Lamp Examination

- The lamp should ideally be allowed to warm up for 1 minute
- The examination room should be perfectly dark
- Light source should be 4 to 5 inches from lesion
- Washing the area before subjecting it to Wood's lamp examination is not permitted
- Topical medicaments, lint and soap residue must be wiped off from site to be examined since these may fluorescence under Wood's lamp.

Applications of Wood's Lamp

- *Superficial fungal infections:*
  - Identification of dermatophyte species capable of producing fluorescence under ultraviolet light. Chemical pteridine is responsible for fluorescence
  - *Malassezia furfur* emits a yellowish-white or copper orange fluorescence.
- *Bacterial infections*
  - *Pseudomonas* produce a pigment pyoverdine which shows green fluorescence under Wood's lamp only if count it is $105/cm^2$
  - *Corynebacterium minutissimum* shows coral red fluorescence under Wood's lamp due to production of water which soluble coproporphyrin III by this bacteria
  - *P. acnes* produces coproporphyrin which imparts orange red fluorescence.
- Demonstration of burrow in scabies by applying fluorescent substances like tetracycline in paste
- Detection of systemize administered drugs, e.g. tetracycline or mepacrine topical tetracycline hydrochloride gives oral red fluorescence which change to yellow after few minutes under Wood's lamp examination.

Water Bath (Fig. 2.26)

Principle: It works on principle of wet heating using convection method of heating. Convection means heated molecules of liquid move up and cooler molecules move to the bottom. Thus setting convection current and keep molecules of fluid moving and mixing well.

Construction

- It consists of two parts: Lid and base, which are made up of steel
- Lid is triangular so that water vapors while forming trickle by the side of inner side of lid back into the base without wetting the contents of base. It prevents heat loss and evaporation
- Base is rectangular box having perforated plate at the bottom
- Base contains at its bottom electric heating coils
- Base is also fitted with thermostat, temperature regulator, off and on switch.

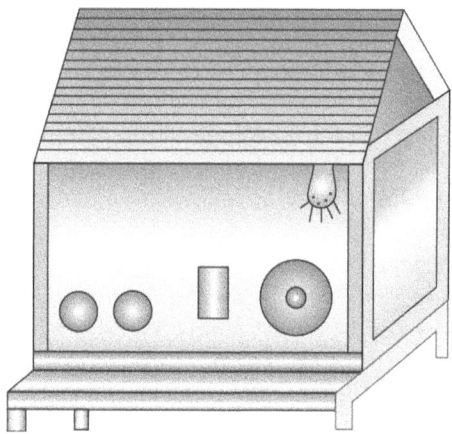

Fig. 2.26: Water bath

Operation

- Keep the required level of water in water bath
- Keep the container containing 1/2 to 2/3rd fluid in such a way that only level of fluid in tubes is dipped in the water of water bath.
- Put the lid at its place over the base and adjust the temperature required
- Put on the switch of water bath
- Note the time when required temperature reaches
- Keep the water bath on till the time, it is required
- Put off the switch before touching water bath.

Precautions

- To avoid electric shock, do not touch the water bath when switch is on
- To keep the fluid molecules in motion make sure that level of water in water bath should be lower than the level of fluid in container (tubes/beaker) being kept in the water bath
- Note the required temperature and then count time for which tubes or beakers or flasks are kept in water bath
- Always keep the lid over base of water bath before putting on the switch.

Uses

- Useful in many serological test where incubation is required, e.g. Widal test

Chapter 2: Laboratory Equipment

- Useful for inactivation of serum
- Solidification or sloping of media may require water bath if inspissator is not available
- Contents of container (e.g. tubes) attain temperature more quicker than incubator.

Distillation Plant (Fig. 2.27)

It is of two types:
1. Single distillation plant
2. Double distillation plant.

Introduction

- This is a process of boiling water
- Then condensing of steam on a cold surface and thus to yielding pure water
- It is electrically heated by a heating coil
- On boiling, the steam is produced which condensed circulating tap water
- The cooled steam is collected and cooled by vessel as distilled water.

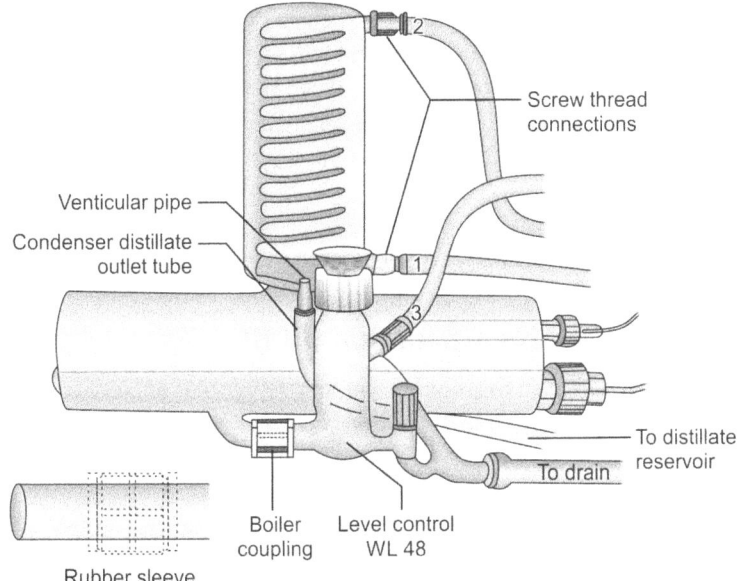

Fig. 2.27: Distillation plant

Procedure

- Make sure that all the water connections are well commuted to the chamber
- Maintain the tap speed for cooling tower faster and the boiling unit slower to prevent unnecessary water overflow
- Switch on the electric supply of both the units and turn on the regulator to a temperature of 100°C
- Make sure that the water levels in both the units are not below the level of heating elements if this stop the concerned unit by switching off the knob or by regulating down the temperature knob
- Leave a container to collect the double distilled water at the output of the second unit
- Once the collecting container is full either stop the unit or replace, if with another empty container to be filled
- In case of any blast or short circuit or leakage immediately turn off the electric and water supply.

Precautions

- Switch off the power in emergency such as power failure and reduction of water supply
- The water still should be regularly cleaned
- Average sized still produce about 4 to 5 liters of water
- Condensed steam is collected in a clean sterile container.

Uses

- Specialized laboratory tests, e.g. enzymes test, distilled water is required
- Distilled water is used for media preparation

Polymerase Chain Reaction (PCR)

It is a technique used to amplify a single or few copies of piece of DNA to generate million of copies of DNA (**Fig. 2.28**).

Principle

It comprises of three steps:
1. DNA extraction from organism by lysis of microorganism and releasing of DNA. It may be done by boiling or using enzyme like lysosomes, etc.

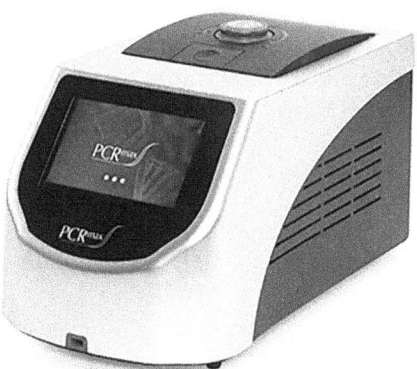

Fig. 2.28: Polymerase chain reaction (PCR) machine

2. Amplification of extracted DNA is done in a machine called thermocycler. The extracted DNA is put to the repeated cycles (30 to 35) of amplification. It is completed in 3 to 4 hours.
   Each amplification has three steps:
   a. Denaturation causing separation of double stranded DNA to different strands. This step is done in 95.
   b. Primer annealing is done in 55. Primer is short oligonucleotides that is complementary site on target ssDNA.
   c. Extension of primer is done at 72. It is done by taq polymerase enzyme. It keeps on adding free nucleotides to the growing end of primer. Taq polymerase is a DNA polymerase from plant bacterium that can withstand high temperature of PCR.
3. Gel electrophoresis of amplified product is done where DNA electrophoretically move according to their molecular size. Now amplified DNA forms clear bands which is seen under ultraviolet light.

Component of PCR

1. DNA template to determine sequence of nucleotide to be amplified
2. Primers:
   - Synthetic strand of about 18 to 25 nucleotides complementary to 3 end of template strand.
   - 2 primers must be present to initiate DNA synthesis.
3. dNTP's (deoxynucleotide triphosphate)
   - Free nucleotide is used as a building block during DNA synthesis

4. DNA polymerase
   - Sequentially adds nucleotides complimentary to template strand at 3-OH bound primers and synthesis new strands of DNA occurs.
   - Commonly used enzyme is Taq polymerase.

Results

- Amplified DNA electrophoretically migrate to their molecular size.
- DNA fragment is seen by staining with ethidium bromide under ultraviolet light.

Application of PCR

1. Genetic testing may detect genetic disease mutation, e.g. sickle cell anemia.
2. Detection of microorganism that is difficult to grow in laboratory.
3. Detects gene in microorganism responsible for drug resistant (*MecA* gene from *Staph*.).
4. Detects little viral genome.
5. Forensic application
6. Research application

Disadvantages

- Conventional PCR detects only DNA however RNA can be detected by reverse transcriptase PCR.
- Conventional PCR can detect presence or absence of DNA however quantity of DNA may be detected using real time PCR.
- PCR cannot differentiate between viable and nonviable organisms.
- False positive amplification may occur due to contamination with environmental DNA. Hence strict asepsis must be obtained in the PCR laboratory.
- PCR inhibitor present in some samples like blood, stools, etc. may inhibit the amplification of target DNA. It may result in false negative result.

Types of PCR

Real Time PCR (rT PCR)

It is used to amplify, detect or quantify a targeted DNA on time bars. Reverse transcriptase in real time PCR format can detect and quantify RNA molecules of test microbes in a sample on Real time bars.

Hence, we use difference thermocycler than conventional PCR.

Advantages of Real Time PCR

- It can quantitate the DNA present in specimen
- It takes less time
- Amplification can be seen simultaneously during process of amplification.
- Contamination rate is quite less.
- Sensitivity and specificity are extremely much higher.

Reverse Transcriptase PCR (RT-PCR)

- Amplify DNA from RNA
- PCR is by reaction rising reverse transcriptase enzyme that converts RNA into DNA
- It is useful for detection of RNA viruses or 16 Sr RNA genes of organisms.

Multiples PCR

- Uses several pairs of primers annealing to different target sequences.
- Permits simultaneous analysis of multiple target in single samples.
- Useful for diagnosis of infectious diseases that are caused by more than one organism. For example, meningitis due to meningococci, pneumococci, *Haemophilus influenzae*.
- Chances of contamination of the reaction tubes do occur with environmental DNA.

Nested PCR

- In this modification of PCR, two rounds of amplification are used. Two primers that are targeted against two different DNA sequence of same microbe.
- It is more sensitive method.
- It is more specific too.
- Nested PCR is useful for detection of *Mycobacterium tuberculosis* (targeting *IS6110* gene) from samples.
- It has disadvantage that the PCR tubes are liable to get contaminated. It may lead to false positive results.

SECTION 2

Human Body Fluids

Section Outline
- ❖ Body Fluids

CHAPTER 3

Body Fluids

EXAMINATION OF URINE

Urine examination is necessary and useful in following ways:
- Finding of functional or structural problems of kidney and urinary tract
- It is also useful to find out diseases like diabetes mellitus (sugar disease), jaundice (liver disease), etc.
- Culture of urine can be done to detect responsible bacteria for urinary tract infection. Culture of urine is also useful to diagnose typhoid fever
- Urine analysis is useful in some metabolic diseases too.

Collection of Urine

- The sample of urine should be examined as early as possible to get best and informative report
- Urine for general examination may be collected in a bottle, properly cleaned with soap and water. It must be properly labeled
- Urine for bacteriological culture should be collected in an autoclaved test tube with cotton swab. Urine should be kept in refrigerator till culture is done
- For culture, midstream urine should be collected
- For routine examination about 100 ml of urine (morning sample) should be collected in a cleaned and dry container
- For the detection of sugar or albumin, urine sample may be collected 2 to 3 hours after meals
- For any quantitative test, specimens of urine may be collected for 24 hours in large bottle. Now amount of sample of urine required can be taken from this 24 hours mixture. This 24 hours collection of urine may also be useful for detection of tubercle bacilli
- In small children, the plastic bag with adhesive mouth fixed around child's genitals for 1 to 3 hours for collection of urine can be used.

Esbach's Albuminometer

It is a graduated glass test tube. It has markings starting from the bottom end as 1, 2, 3, etc., U and R. The digits 1, 2, 3, etc. indicate the proteins in grams per liter of urine. The marking U is for filling the urine up to the level, R is for the Esbach's reagent. The albuminometer stands vertical in a wooden base. A wooden cover, is for the safety of the glass tube. The mouth of the tube is closed with a rubber cork (**Fig. 3.1**).

Procedure

Fill the urine in the albuminometer up to the mark U. Add Esbach's reagents until the mark 'R'. Cork the albuminometer. Mix urine with the reagent by gently inverting the albuminometer several times. Allow it to stand upright for 10 to 12 hours (overnight). Read the level of the yellow precipitate of proteins next day as grams of albumin (proteins) per liter of urine.

Preservation of Urine Specimen

- Urine may be preserved if quantitative examination is to be done
- Urine sample can be kept in refrigerator

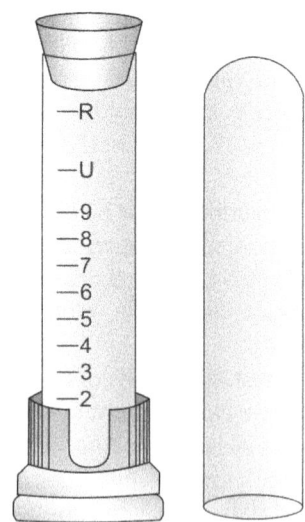

Fig. 3.1: Esbach's albuminometer

- Preservatives used are:
  - Toluol (2 ml per 100 ml of urine)
  - Thymol
  - Formalin (1 drop per 30 ml of urine)
  - Boric acid (0.3 gm per 120 ml of urine).

Routine Examination of Urine

Physical Examination

Volume

- Average urine passed out by adult in 24 hours is 1200 to 1500 ml
- During night, urine quantity is never more than 400 ml.

Odor

- It is recorded in fresh urine sample only
- If ketone bodies are present, then the odor of urine is fruity
- In the presence of certain bacteria, urine is of ammoniacal odor.

Color

- Look for the color of urine. It may be colorless, yellow, dark yellow, brown, blood stained (red color). Also observe whether urine is clear or turbid (cloudy).

Specific Gravity

- Measure the specific gravity with an instrument called urinometer. Calibration of urinometer is 1.000 (specific gravity of water) to 1.050. Concentrated urine has high specific gravity and diluted urine has low specific gravity. Specific gravity of urine is measured as (**Figs 3.2A to E**):
  - Take 40 ml of urine into a measuring cylinder
  - Lower the urinometer gently into the urine and leave it as such
  - Wait for sometime so that urinometer settles
  - Read off the specific gravity given on the scale at the surface of the urine (lowest point of meniscus)
  - Normal specific gravity of urine is 1.0 to 1.025
  - Low specific gravity is there in kidney and endocrine diseases
  - High specific gravity is due to presence of high protein and sugar in urine.

Section 2: Human Body Fluids

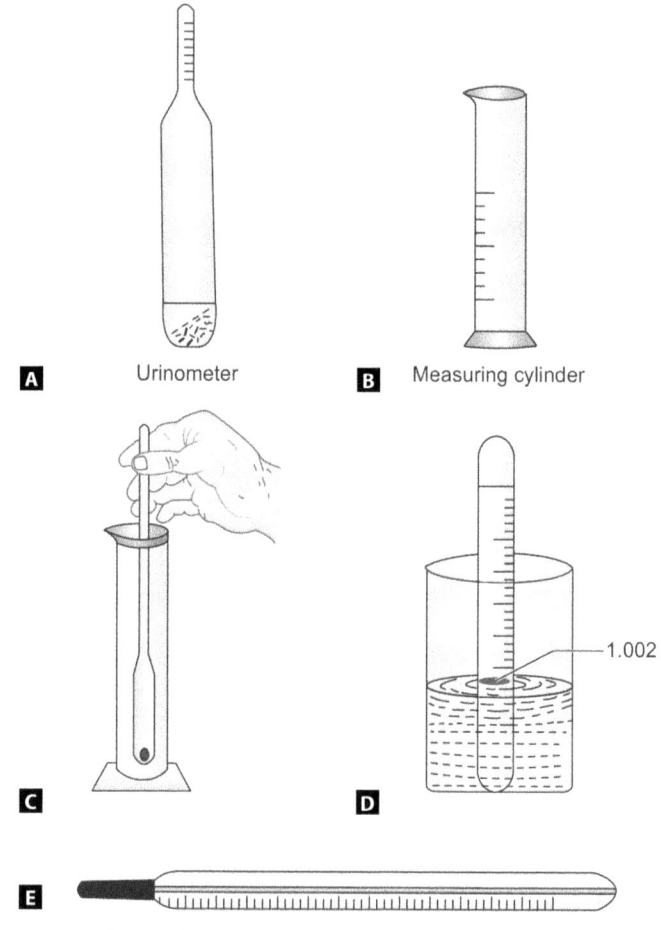

Figs 3.2A to E: Measurement of specific gravity of urine

Urinometer

Construction

The instrument to determine specific gravity of urine is called urinometer. It is made of glass. It has a bulb-like lower end usually filled with mercury or some heavy material. It is followed by a bigger bulb usually empty. The third part is a narrow tube, graduated from 1000 to 1050 equal divisions and closed at the top (**Fig. 3.2A**).

A wide- mouthed cylinder is usually supplied with the urinometer (**Fig. 3.2B**). The graduation reads the specific gravity of the urine at a certain temperature, which is engraved on the urinometer.

Procedure

Fill the cylinder to about 2/3 height. Allow the urinometer to float freely in the urine (**Fig. 3.2C**). The urinometer should not touch the sides of the cylinder or the bottom. Read the graduation mark on the urinometer which coincides with the surface of urine. Check the zero of the instrument by taking specific gravity of distilled water. This should read zero. Note the temperature of the urine sample (**Fig. 3.2D**). For every 3°C temperature above the temperature marked on the urinometer, subtract 1 division. For temperature of the urine below the marked temperature add 1 division for every 3°C to get the correct specific gravity (**Fig. 3.2E**).

pH of Urine

It is normally of acidic (pH 6.0) measured as under:
- Place in a watch glass 1 strip of universal indicator paper (pH 1 to 10)
- Place few drops of urine on the paper
- Pick-up the strip of paper with forceps. Compare the color obtained with those shown on standard chart
- Read off and note down the pH reading given for color most closely matching the test paper
- Now select a strip indicator paper for corresponding range of pH, e.g. for pH reading 8, select indicator paper of range 6 to 8
- Repeat the test in another glass watch using selected indicator paper.

Alternatively, pH reading can also be taken by dipping the indicator paper directly into urine sample.

Normal pH = 5.0 to 7.0

Acidic pH (4.5 to 5.5) occurs in diabetes mellitus (sugar disease), tired muscles, etc.

Alkaline pH (7.8 to 8) usually seen in urinary tract infection.

Normally, the pH of a mixed 24 hours urine is around 6. Urine turns alkaline on standing due to ammoniacal fermentation.

It becomes alkaline due to:
- Infection
- Severe vomiting
- High intake of fruits and vegetables
- Alkaline therapy

Urine becomes acidic in:
- Pyelonephritis
- Tuberculosis of kidney
- Acidosis
- Muscular exercises
- High protein
- On fasting.

Chemical Examination

Glucose

Detection of glucose in urine is done as under:
- Pipette 5 ml of Benedict solution into a test tube
- Boil it over spirit lamp
- Add 8 drops (0.5 ml) of urine and mix well
- Boil over spirit lamp for 2 minutes
- Leave the mixture to cool to room temperature and examine the color change of mixture.

Color	Result %
Blue	Negative
Green	A trace
Green with yellow precipitate	+ 0.5%
Yellow to dark green	++ 1%
Orange	+++ 1.5%
Brick red	++++2%

Nowadays reagent strips are also available for detection of sugar in urine sample.

Protein

Detection of protein in urine is done as under :
- Fill the test tube about two-thirds with urine
- Hold the test tube at an angle to flame. It is done to boil only the upper layer of urine in test tube
- If urine becomes turbid (cloudy), then add a few drops of acetic acid (5%) to it. In normal urine, cloudiness disappears
- Boil the urine again. If cloudiness remains as such it means protein (albumin) is present.

No cloudiness	Protein negative
Slight cloudy urine	+
Heavy cloudiness	(++), and above expressed as +++, ++++

Bile Pigments

Detection of bile pigments in urine may be using Lugol's iodine test as under:
- Put 4 ml of urine in a test tube
- Add 4 drops of Lugol's iodine in the urine
- Shake the tube and note down the color which is produced at once.

Negative test	Faint yellow color
Positive test	Pale green color + Deep green color ++

Bile pigment detection can also be done by another test called Fouchet's test. It is done as under:
- Take 5 ml of urine in a test tube and add 2.5 ml of barium chloride
- After mixing precipitates are formed
- Filter the mixture. The precipitates containing bile remain on the filter paper. Spread the filter paper on another dry filter paper to remove excess of water
- Add 2 drops of Fouchet's reagent to the precipitate on the filter paper. The color of precipitate changes to green or blue if bile pigments are present.

Bile Salts

Detection of bile salt is done as under by Hay's sulfur powder test:
- Cool the urine by placing it in a cool place
- Add some urine in a wide test tube or small beaker
- Sprinkle finely powdered sulfur on the surface of urine
- *Negative test*: Sulfur flowers float on the surface of urine
  Positive test: Sulfur flowers sink to the bottom.

Ketone Bodies

Detection of ketone bodies may be done as under:
- Place few crystals of sodium nitroprusside in a test tube and add 5 ml of distilled water. Shake well till crystals are almost dissolved.

Some crystals must remain undissolved at the bottom of tube. It is a saturated solution
- In a test tube take 5 to 10 ml of urine
- Add enough of solid ammonium sulfate with shaking to make a saturated solution
- Now add 2 to 3 drops of freshly prepared sodium nitroprusside solution (saturated)
- Mix well
- Add about 1 ml of liquor ammonia slowly on to the surface of mixture with pipette
- *Negative test*: No change in color
 Positive test: Purple ring at the junction of two layers.

Blood in Urine

Blood in urine may be detected as under:
- Microscopic examination of urinary sediments
- Spectroscopic examination of urine for blood absorption bands
- *Chemical tests*:
  - Take about 2 ml of urine in a test tube
  - Add about 1.0 ml of benzidine solution (saturated) in acetic acid
  - Mix and add 4 to 5 drops of hydrogen peroxide (100 vol%)
  - The mixture develops peacock blue color if blood is present.

Microscopic Examination

Microscopic examination is done as under:
- Mix the urine gently
- Put the urine in centrifuge tube till it is 3/4 full
- Centrifuge at about 2500 revolutions per minute (RPM) for 5 minutes
- Pour off the fluid by inverting the tube without shaking
- Now shake the deposit with the remaining 1 to 2 drops of urine
- Put one drop on clean glass slide and cover it with coverslip
- Number the slide with the number of specimen
- Examine the slide under microscope using first 10X objective and then 40X objective. Keep the condenser lowered to make transparent things visible.

Now look for the following things under microscope:
1. *Erythrocytes* (red blood cells) which may be seen as:
   - Small yellowish disc which is darker at the edge about 8 µ in diameter. This RBC is intact (**Fig. 3.3A**).

- Spiky-edged small size (5 to 6 μ) is a crenated RBC (**Fig. 3.3B**)
- Thin, circle, large sized (9 to 10 μ) are swollen RBC (**Fig. 3.3C**).

2. *Leukocytes* (white blood cells) are seen as:
   - Clear, granular disc, 10 to 15 μ in intact leukocyte (**Fig. 3.3D**)
   - Shrunken, less granular and distorted shape, in degenerated leukocyte (**Fig. 3.3E**)
   - Clumps of many degenerated cells in case of pus (**Fig. 3.3F**)
   - Presence of many white cells in clumps means infection of urinary tract.
3. *Yeasts* are seen (**Fig. 3.3G**) as:
   - Round or oval structure
   - Budding may be seen
   - Yeasts are of various sizes.
4. *Trichomonas* (**Fig. 3.3H**) look as under:
   - 15 μ in size
   - Round or globular in shape
   - Moves in fresh urine
   - Organs of movement are flagella which are 4 in number
   - Undulating membrane like a fin of fish may be seen on one side only.
5. *Spermatozoa* may be seen (**Fig. 3.3I**) in urine of male:
   - Head is 5 μ
   - Flagellum is very long (50 μ)
   - Show active movements in fresh urine.
6. *Epithelial cells* (**Fig. 3.3J**) may be of following types:
   - *Squamous epithelial cells*
     - Large rectangular
     - They may come from urethra or vagina.
   - *Bladder cells*
     - Diamond-shaped large cells with nucleus.
   - *Cells from pelvis of kidney*
     - Medium size cells
     - Granular
     - There is a short tail.
   - *Cells from ureter and pelvis of kidney*:
     - Medium-sized oval cell with nucleus
     - If they are many with leukocytes and filaments, they may be from ureter

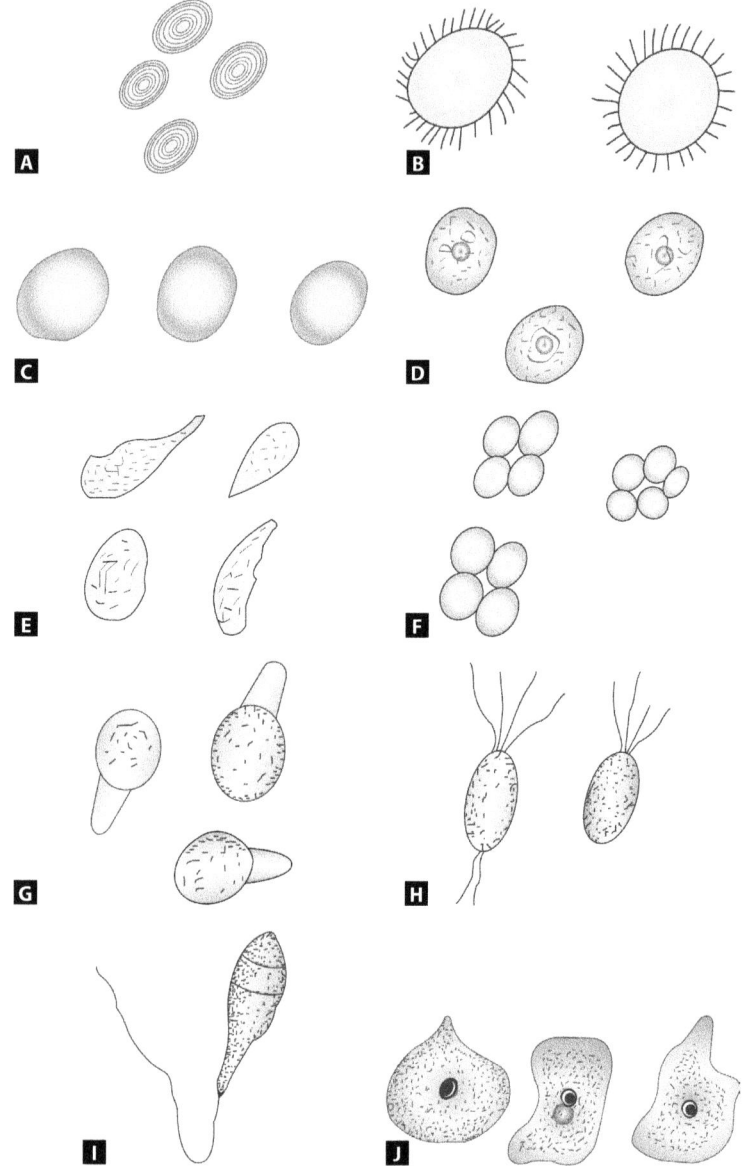

Figs 3.3A to J: (A) Intact red blood cells; (B) Crenated red blood cells; (C) Swollen red blood cells; (D) Intact white blood cells; (E) Shrunken white blood cells; (F) Pus cells; (G) Yeast cells; (H) *Trichomonas*; (I) Spermatozoa; (J) Squamous epithelial cells

- If they are few with no leukocytes, then they may be pelvic cells.
- *Renal cells* are:
  - Small
  - Very granular
  - They are always present with protein in urine.
7. *Casts* are of following features:
   - Cylindrical in shape and long
   - Cross almost the whole field when examined under microscope using 40X objective
   - Casts may be of following types:
     - *Hyaline cast* (**Fig. 3.4A**)
       i. Transparent and refractile
       ii. Ends are rounded or tapered
       iii. May be found in healthy person after heavy exercise.
     - *Fine granular casts* (**Fig. 3.4B**)
       i. Granules are smaller and do not fill the cast.
     - *Blood casts* (**Fig. 3.4C**)
       i. Brown in color
       ii. Casts are filled with degenerated RBC.
     - *Pus casts* (**Fig. 3.4D**)
       i. Cast is fully filled with degenerated leukocytes.
     - *Epithelial casts* (**Fig. 3.4E**)
       i. Cast is filled with pale yellow epithelial cells.
     - *Fatty acids casts (rare)*
       i. Very refractile
       ii. Ends rounded and edges indented
       iii. Found in severe kidney diseases
       iv. Soluble in ether.
8. *Crystals* may be of following types (**Figs 3.5A to G**):
   - *Calcium oxalate* (**Fig. 3.5A**)
     - Shape is like an envelope
     - Size is 10 to 20 μ.
   - *Uric acid* (**Fig. 3.5B**)
     - Shape may be like square, diamond, cubical or rose
     - 30 to 150 μ in size
     - Yellow or brownish red in color.

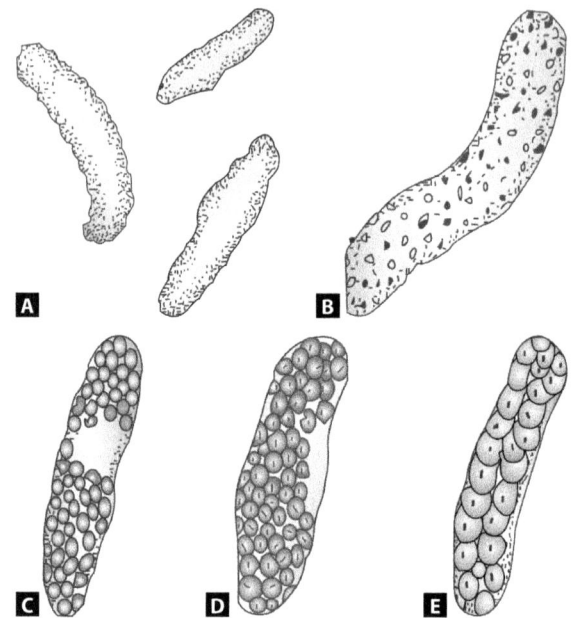

Figs 3.4A to E: (A) Hyaline; (B) Granular; (C) Blood cast; (D) Pus cast; (E) Epithelial cast

- *Triple phosphate* (**Fig. 3.5C**)
    - Found in alkaline or neutral pH urine
    - Rectangular or star shaped
    - 30 to 150 μ in size
    - Colorless and refractile.
- *Urates*
    - Present in acidic urine
    - Like bundle or needles
    - 20 μ in size
    - Color is yellow
    - Refractile.

Other crystals seen in urine less oftenly are:
- Calcium phosphate (star-shaped)
- Calcium carbonate (millet grains grouped in pairs)
- Calcium sulfate (long prism like)
- Cystine (hexagonal)
- Cholesterol (squarish plates with notch on one side)
    - Bilirubin (tiny crystals, square or like heads or needles).

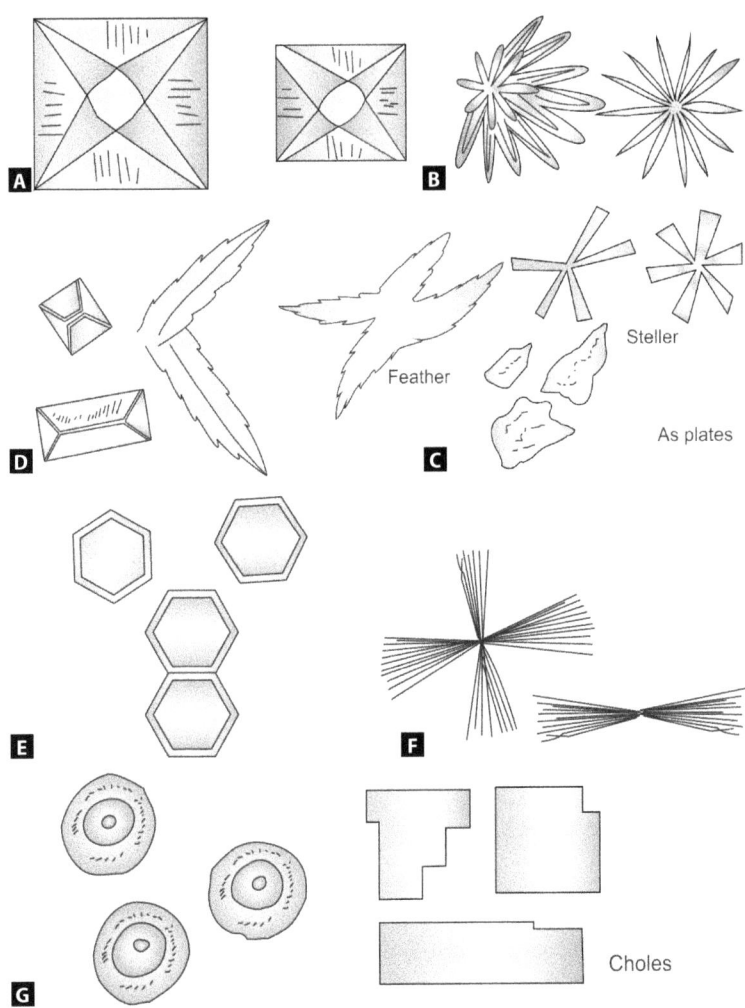

Figs 3.5A to G: Crystals Cholesterol. (A) Calcium oxalate; (B) Uric acid; (C) Triple phosphate; (D) Calcium hydrogen phosphate; (E) Cystine; (F) Tyrosine; (G) Leucine

EXAMINATION OF CEREBROSPINAL FLUID (CSF)

Functions of CSF

Cerebrospinal fluid is formed by choroid plexus of ventricles of brain. It protects the brain and spinal cord from external pressure injuries. It also provides nutrients thus acting as a nutrient medium. It is involved in excreting waste products of metabolism of nervous tissue.

Features of CSF

- *Colors*: CSF is clear, colorless fluid
- *Volumes*: Total volume in adult is 100 to 150 ml
- *Specific gravity*: Specific gravity is 1.006 to 1.008
- *Reaction*: Alkaline in reaction.

Collection of Specimen

- CSF is collected by puncturing the space between 3rd and 4th lumbar vertebrae. It is called lumbar puncture. Specimen collection may be done by expert doctor under sterilized conditions
- About 3 to 5 ml of CSF can be collected in 3 tubes (5 ml each)
- It is sent immediately to the laboratory for tests.

Physical Examination

- Normally CSF is crystal clear.
- Color of CSF is changed in diseases. Presence of blood (reddish) in CSF may mean bleeding (subarachnoid or intraventricular haemorrhage). It may be yellow tinged. e.g. in jaundice. A cloudy or turbid fluid may mean brain abscess, bacterial infection of covering of brain (meningitis). A fine pellicle of clot in fluid is found in tuberculosis of meninges.

Cytological Examination

Leukocyte (WBC) count: It should done immediately after collection of CSF as described here:
- Draw Unna's polychrome methylene blue to mark 1 in a RBC pipette and fill pipette up to mark 101 with CSF
- The reagent colors red cell yellow and white cells blue
- Cover the counting chamber (Neubauer) with coverslip and put a drop of fluid and allow the fluid to spread under the coverslip
- Wait for 1 to 5 minutes to settle cells.
- Count 9 large squares in counting chamber for both RBCs and WBCs
- The total cells counted multiplied by 1.1 gives the number of cells per cu mm.

Differential count : Centrifuge the CSF and make smears from deposits and stain by Leishman's stain. Count about 100 or more cells and record the percentage (%) of cells. A large number of lymphocytes are observed in tuberculosis whereas large number of segmented leukocytes are seen in bacterial meningitis.

Gram's staining: Staining the smear by Gram's method shows whether bacteria are gram-positive (violet color) or gram-negative (red color).

Ziehl-Neelsen stained smears: Staining the smear by Ziehl-Neelsen method shows whether acid-fast bacilli (tubercular bacteria) are present or absent.

Papanicolaou staining: Tumor's cells (cancer cells) may be seen by using Papanicolaou stain.

Chemical Examination

Estimation of Total Protein

Normal value is 15-45 mg%
- Take 1 ml of the CSF in a tube
- Add 3 ml of 3% sulfosalicylic acid
- Mix and allow the mixture to stand for 5 minutes
- Significant turbidity if present, means presence of increased protein
- Compare the turbidity in a colorimeter with standard.

Qualitative Tests for Increase in Globulin

Pandy's Test

- Take 1 ml solution of carbolic acid (10 gm + 150 ml water) in a Kahn's tube or Wassermann's tube
- Add to it one drop of CSF
- No change in normal CSF
- If globulin is in excess, then bluish ring develops.

Nonne-Apelt Test

- Take 1 ml of saturated ammonium sulfate solution in a test tube
- 1 ml of CSF is layered over it
- Allow it to stand for 3 minutes
- A white or gray ring at the point of contact indicates excess of globulin.

Sugar Estimation

- Normal value is 45 to 70 mg%
- Increased values are observed in diabetes mellitus, uremia, brain tumor, etc.
- Decreased values are seen in acute meningitis (30 mg%), tuberculosis meninges (6 to 40 mg%), etc.
- Quantitative estimation of sugar may be done by o-toluidine method as in blood sugar estimation
- Remember that tests for sugar must always be done on freshly collected CSF.

Chloride Estimation

- Normal value for adults is 720 to 760 mg% and for children, it is 625 to 670 mg%
- Decreased levels are seen in tuberculosis of meninges
- Levels remain normal in tumors, brain abscess, etc.
- Increased values are seen in hypertension.

Silver Nitrate Titration Method

Principle

Chloride presents in the CSF is directly titrated with silver nitrate.
$$AgNO_3 + NaCl \rightarrow AgCl + NaNO_3$$
When chloride ions are exhausted, the excess silver ions react with chromate ions to form red solution of silver chromate.
$$2AgNO_3 + K_2CrO_4 \rightarrow Ag_2CrO_4/(red\ precipitates) + 2KNO_3$$

Reagents

- Silver nitrate solution 25 mEq/L (4.25 g/L) check against sodium chloride 125 mEq/L (7.3125 gm/liter). 1 ml of this should require exactly 5 ml of silver nitrate
- Potassium chromate 10%.

Procedures

Take about 30 ml water in a small beaker or 28 mm × 150 mm test tube. Add 1 ml CSF followed by 2 to 3 drops of potassium chromate. Mixture is titrated with silver nitrate solution to a faint brick of red color. Normal fluid requires about 5 ml of silver nitrate.

Calculation

CSF chloride (mEq/L) = ml of silver nitrate solution used × 25.

Bacteriological Examination

- *Culture in 10% CO_2*
    - Cloudy fluid should be cultured on chocolate agar (bacterial), Sabouraud's agar (fungi), nutrient agar, blood broth and thioglycollate media. Incubation is done at 37°C in candle jar to provide 10% CO_2
    - Sediments of centrifuged fluid should be cultured on Löwenstein-Jensen media to grow tubercle bacilli, if present
    - Guinea pig injection of CSF in peritoneal cavity may be useful for the diagnosis of tuberculosis
- *Serological test*
    - Wassermann test (complement fixation test)
    - Kahn's test
    - VDRL test
    - Latex agglutination and CFT for fungal infection (cryptococcal infection).

Reporting of Cerebrospinal Fluid Examination

- *Physical examination*
    - Color
    - Transparency
    - Clot formation (Cobweb)
    - Pressure
- *Cytological examination*
    - Total cell count
    - Predominant cells
- *Staining*
    - Leishman's stain
    - Gram's staining
    - Ziehl-Neelsen stain
    - Papanicolaou stain
- *Chemical examination*
    - Proteins
        i. Total protein
        ii. Qualitative globulin

- Sugar value
- Chloride value
* Microbiological examination
  - Culture of bacteria
  - Culture of tubercle bacilli
  - Culture for fungi
  - Animal inoculation (Guinea pig and mice)
  - Serological tests.

STOOL EXAMINATION

Stool examination is important as it provides many informations including demonstration of ova, cysts, parasites (helminths), disease-causing bacteria, etc.

Collection of Stool

It is done as under:
* Stool should be collected in sufficient quantity
* Stool must be collected in a proper container, e.g. waxed cardboard box, a wide-mouthed plastic bottle with a lid (**Figs 3.6A and B**), etc.
* Stool should be sent and processed in the laboratory within 1 hour of its passing by the patient

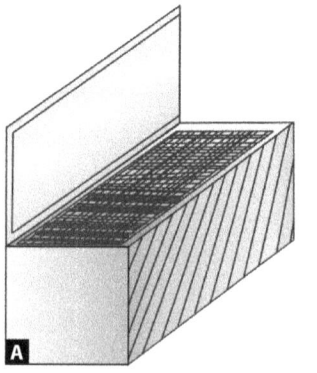
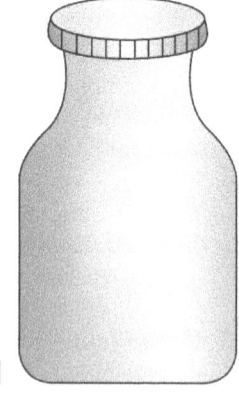

Figs 3.6A and B: Containers for stool collection. (A) Waxed cardboard; (B) Wide-mouthed plastic bottle with lid

- For cholera bacilli study, it may be collected in transport media, e.g. alkaline peptone water
- For parasites (ova/cyst), stool should be collected in 30 ml bottle containing 15 ml of 10% formaldehyde solution.

Physical Examination

- Quantity of stool should be at least 4 ml
- Note the consistency, e.g. firm, hard, soft, watery, etc.
- Color should be recorded, e.g. light to dark brown, black, clay colored, etc.
- Also note the other features, e.g. mucus, blood, streaks of pus, worm or segment of worm, etc.

Chemical Examination

Blood in Stools (Benzidine Test)

- Mix stool with about 5 ml water in a test tube
- Add 2 ml of benzidine solution (saturated) in glacial acetic acid
- Mix well and add 1 ml of 30% hydrogen peroxide
- A deep blue color means test is positive. It means blood is present in stool.

Microscopic Examination

Slide Preparation

- Mark the number of specimen on slide with grease pencil
- *Place on the slide*:
  - One drop of normal saline in the middle of left half of slide
  - One drop of Lugol's iodine in the middle of the right half of the slide.
- Take small quantity of stool with a wireloop
- Mix it with a drop of normal saline on the slide
- Likewise take again small quantity of stool and mix it with the drop of Lugol's iodine
- Place a coverslip over each drop.
- Examine the preparation as under:
  - For saline preparation, use 10X and 40X objectives and 5X eyepiece. Keep the condenser low
  - For iodine preparation, use 40X objective.

Concentration Method Using Saturated Sodium Chloride Solution

- Place a portion of stool (2 ml) in a cleaned penicillin bottle
- Add small quantity of saturated sodium chloride solution to fill 1/4th of bottle. Mix the stool
- Now fill the bottle to the top with saturated sodium chloride solution
- Remove anything which floats
- Place a coverslip carefully over the mouth of bottle
- Coverslip must be in contact with liquid mixture of the bottle
- Wait for 20 to 30 minutes
- Lift the coverslip carefully in such a way that a drop of liquid should remain on the slide
- Coverslip is kept over the drop of liquid
- Study it under microscope for eggs.

Microscopic examination may show following:

Protozoa

- *Entamoeba histolytica* (**Fig. 3.7A**)
- *Entamoeba coli* (**Fig. 3.7B**)
- *Giardia lamblia* (**Fig. 3.7C**)
- *Balantidium coli* (**Fig. 3.7D**).

Helminths (Eggs/Ova)

- *Ascaris lumbricoides* (roundworm) (**Fig. 3.8A**)
- *Ancylostoma duodenale* (hookworm) (**Fig. 3.8B**)
- *Enterobius vermicularis* (pinworm) (**Fig. 3.8C**)
- *Trichuris trichiura* (whipworm) (**Fig. 3.8D**).

Miscellaneous

Bacteriological Examination

- Direct smear for the demonstration of tubercle bacilli (acid-fast bacilli). *Vibrio cholerae* may be seen in epithelia cells as gram-negative (red color and curved comma-shaped bacilli)
- Hanging drop preparation is used to demonstrate darting motility of *Vibrio cholerae*
- Culture is done to identify bacteria causing diseases like typhoid, diarrhea and dysentery.

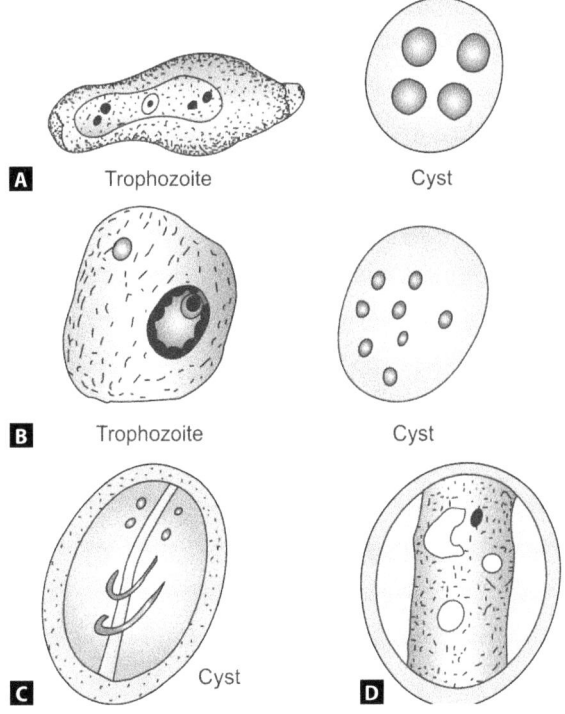

Figs 3.7A to D: Protozoa

EXAMINATION OF SPUTUM

Sputum is a material of lungs, bronchi and larynx. Its examination is useful to find diseases causing bacteria, fungi, parasites, viruses, etc. Sputum examination is helpful in finding cancer cells in a patient of lungs cancer.

Collection of Sputum Specimen

- Patient should rinse the mouth with water before coughing out specimen
- Collect the sputum in the morning
- Sputum must be collected in glass screw top jars or waxed paper cup (ice-cream **Fig. 3.9**) with lid

Section 2: Human Body Fluids

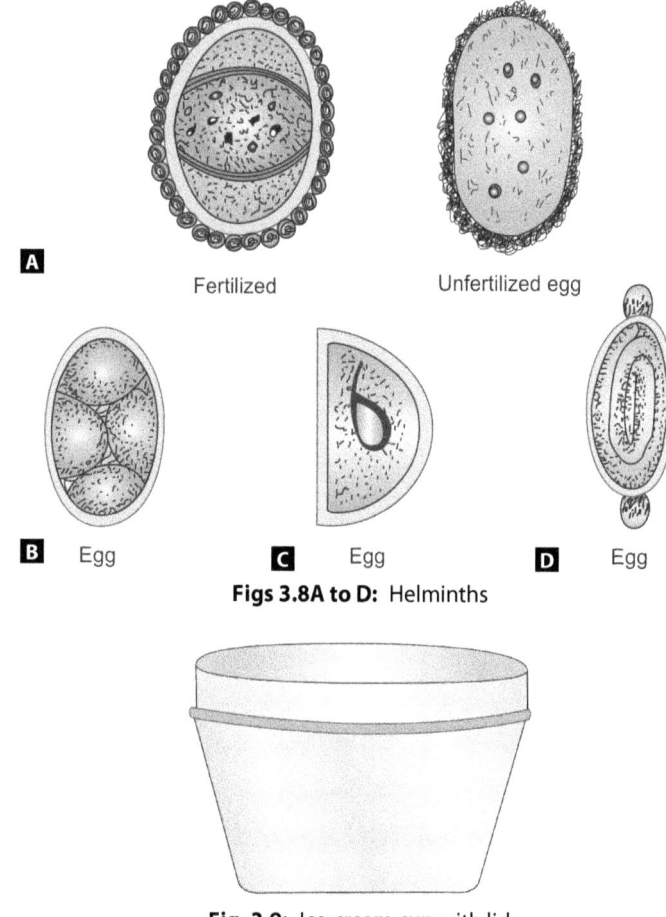

Figs 3.8A to D: Helminths

Fig. 3.9: Ice-cream cup with lid

- After collection of sputum specimen, write the name of the patient, date of collection and specimen number.

Physical Examination
- *Quantity*
  - Small
  - Moderate
  - Large

- *Consistency*
  - Frothy
  - Mucoid and thick
  - Blood stained
  - Pus containing
  - Thin and watery
- *Smell*
  - Smellness
  - Foul smelling
- *Color*
  - Colorless
  - Whitish yellow or greenish (pus)
  - Blackish (carbon particles)
  - Bright red colored stained (fresh blood)
  - Dark brown (old blood).

Microscopic Examination

- *Preparation of sputum smear*
  - With glass marking pencil, write the specimen number on slide
  - Keep wireloop over spirit-lamp flame till it becomes red hot
  - Cool the wireloop and take thick sputum
  - Place it over the slide and move the wireloop in an oval spiral outwards from the center (**Fig. 3.10**)
  - Make smear and allow smear to dry in the air
  - Dip the loop in Lysol solution and keep the loop over spirit-lamp flame to make it red hot.
- *Examination of unstained sputum*
  It may be done for followings:
  - Charcot-Leyden crystal which are colorless, needle-shaped crystals
  - Calcified nodules are stones which may be small in size
  - Myelin globules are seen as colorless and pear shaped

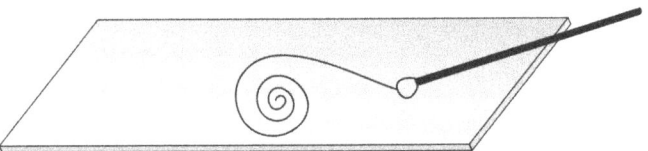

Fig. 3.10: Preparation of sputum smear

- Parasites may be seen in the form of hooklets of hydatid disease. In case of liver abscess involving lung (by getting ruptured), it may be possible to see trophozoites of *Entamoeba histolytica*
- Fungi are seen as rounded (yeast), elongated round (budding yeast cells) or thread-like (hyphae) structures.
- *Examination of stained smear*
  - Leishman stained smears may show epithelial cells, white blood cells, bacteria or thread like structures
  - For cancer cell demonstration proceed as under:
    i. Spread fresh sputum on glass dish
    ii. Tease out fragment on a glass slide. Prepare six such slides
    iii. Dip slides in Schaudinn's solution (SS) (10 ml absolute alcohol + 20 ml SS mercuric chloride + 3% glacial acetic acid) for 20 minutes
    iv. Wash the slides for 2 minutes in alcoholic iodine. Alcoholic iodine contains 2% iodine 20 ml (2 Vols). Absolute alcohol 40 ml (4 Vols)
    v. Now wash the slides with distilled water
    vi. Stain with hematoxylin and eosin (H and E) and after mounting study under microscope for cancer cells
    vii. Papanicolaou method is also useful for finding out cancer cell in fresh sputum specimen
  - Gram's staining may be helpful in finding bacteria, like Pneumococci, *Streptococcus pyogenes, Staphylococcus aureus*, etc.
  - Ziehl-Neelsen stained smear is helpful in finding tubercle bacilli.

Reporting of Sputum

It is done as under:

Physical Examination

- Quantity
- Consistency
- Smell
- Color
- Pus
- Blood

Microscopic Examination

- Wet unstained preparation
- Stained preparation like H and E, Ziehl-Neelsen, Gram's and Leishman's stain

Culture of Sputum

- It may be done to identify bacteria and finding out effective antibacterial drugs
- Culture can also be done to find out and identifying bacteria, fungi or viruses.

EXAMINATION OF SEMEN

Semen is formed by testes present only in males. Semen consists of spermatozoa and seminal plasma. Semen examination is done in patient of sterility. The cause of male sterility may be defective spermatozoa or number of spermatozoa is quite less. Semen examination is also done in persons who are operated upon vasectomy, to check that spermatozoa are present in the semen.

Collection of Semen

- Patient should be asked not to pass semen for about 2 to 5 days, before test
- Patient is asked to discharge semen using his hand (masturbation)
- Specimen of semen may be collected in clean and dry tube
- Specimen should reach laboratory for examination within 15 minutes.
- Note the date, time of collection and time of receiving specimen
- Examine semen only after liquefaction (30 to 60 minutes).

Physical Examination

Volume
- Measure the volume of semen in graduated cylinder
- Normal volume is 2 to 5 ml.

Color
- Normal semen is opaque, white or grayish in color
- Normal semen does not contain blood, pus or mucus.

Consistency
- Note down the consistency of specimen at the time of receiving it
- Find out the time taken for the semen to become liquid

- Fresh semen when passed out is viscid and clot quickly. It liquefies within 20 to 60 minutes.

pH

- Dip a strip of pH indicator paper (pH between 6 and 8) in the semen and read the pH given for the color most closely matching the test paper
- Normal pH ranges from 7 to 7.7.

Microscopic Examination

Sperm Motility

- Sperm motility is seen at room temperature
- Place a drop of semen on a clean glass slide
- Cover the drop with a coverslip
- Apply vaseline at the edge of coverslip to prevent drying
- Examine the slide under microscope under 10X objective
- When sperms are seen, shift to 40X objective
- Remember that light is reduced by adjusting iris diaphragm
- Count number of actively motile, sluggishly motile and non-motile sperms among 100 sperms. Normally, sperms are:
  – Actively motile   80%
  – Sluggishly motile or non-motile   20%

Sperm Count

- Pipette 0.95 ml of diluting fluid into a small bottle using 1 ml of graduated pipette
- Draw well mixed semen with WBC pipette up to 0.05 ml mark
- Blow 0.05 ml of semen into bottle containing 0.95 ml of diluting fluid (1:20 dilution)
- Mix the contents well
- Keep coverslip properly over Neubauer chamber
- Add diluted semen with the help of pipette, by the side of coverslip
- Leave this chamber for 3 minutes on the bench. By this time, sperm will settle down
- Count the number of sperm in one large corner square (area of 1 mm^2). Use 10X objective and 6X eyepiece
- While counting sperm, consider only complete sperms with intact heads and tails.

Calculation
　　Number of sperms in one large square = A
　　Number of sperms per ml = A × 200000 millions.

Example
Number of sperms counted = 400
Sperms count = 400 × 200000 = 80 millions/ml
Normal sperm count = 60 to 150 millions/ml

Sperm Morphology

- Allow liquefaction of semen in ½ to 1 hour.
- Draw a smear of semen on a clean glass slide (like thin blood smear).
- Dry the smear in air.
- Fix the smear by passing it quickly over a flame once or twice.
- Cool the slide and cover the smear with 25% aqueous basic fuchsin. Keep it up for 5 minutes.
- Wash with tap water and dry the smeared slide.
- Examine the slide under oil immersion
- Count all sperms in the field
- Count defective sperms
- Change field and count a total of 100 sperms and report:
　　Normal sperms = %
　　Defective sperms = %

(Defective sperms, should not be more than 20% in healthy man, **Figs 3.11A and B**).

Other Cells

Also study other cells in semen like:
- Red blood cells
- White blood cells
- Epithelial cells.

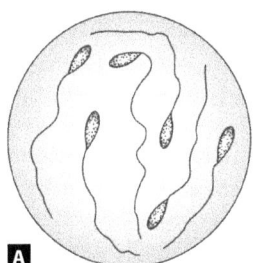
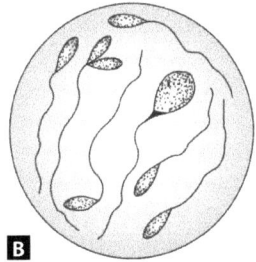

Figs 3.11A and B: Spermatozoa (A) Normal and (B) Abnormal

SECTION 3

Microbiology

Section Outline
- ❖ Microbiology

Microbiology

BACTERIOLOGY

Microbiology

Microbiology is the branch of science that deals with the study of viruses, and bacteria, fungi and parasites which cannot be seen through naked eyes.

Bacteriology

Bacteriology deals with the study of bacteria.

Bacteria

Bacteria are microscopic, single-celled structures which re-produce by dividing into two by a process called binary fission. Bacteria are of many types. They may be found in soil, air, water and in food. Some of them may live on skin and in the body of man.

Many bacteria do useful work, making the animals and plants to live. For example, there are bacteria in the soil, helping to make the soil fertile by producing nitrates from nitrogen in the air. Some bacteria are necessary for man, such as those which live in his intestine helping to break food material, produce vitamins and prevent attack by harmful bacteria.

In medical microbiology, the organisms we are concerned with, are disease producing bacteria.

Transmission of Bacteria

Transmission of bacteria occurs:
- By eating bacteria containing food thus causing dysentery, typhoid fever, etc.
- By drinking water containing bacteria, e.g. cholera.
- Through roadside accidental wounds, e.g. tetanus.

- By using unsterilized bacteria containing instruments like scissors, knife, syringes, needles, etc.
- By breathing in of bacteria containing air in overcrowded houses, e.g. tuberculosis.
- By bites of insects, e.g. bubonic plague.
- By scratching the bites produced by insects like louse-borne typhus, eczema, etc.
- By direct contact from person to person, e.g. gonorrhea, syphilis, etc.

How do Disease Causing Bacteria Produce Disease?

- The bacteria in high number have better chances of producing disease.
- If person is weak, his chances of having disease produced by bacteria are more. Such person cannot fight with attacking bacteria and killing them.
- The bacteria produce disease by multiplying rapidly and damaging the cells of body.
- Production of toxin by bacteria inside the body can cause disease.

Laboratory Identification of Bacteria

- By examining the bacteria directly under the microscope to know the shape, size, motility, arrangement (pair, cluster or chain), etc.
- By examining the bacteria in a stained specimen.
- By culturing, i.e. growing the organisms, using what is known as culture media.
- Identification of cultured bacteria with the help of biochemical reactions.

Types of Specimens Received in Bacteriology Laboratory

Urine: For bacteria causing urinary tract infection
Stool: For bacteria which may produce dysentery, diarrhea, typhoid, fever, etc.
Sputum: For bacteria causing lung infection like pneumonia, tuberculosis.
Cerebrospinal fluid: For bacteria which may cause infection of brain layer called meninges (meningitis).
Blood: For bacteria which may enter the blood (Bacteremia).
Aspirates: For bacteria producing pus, e.g. abscess

Fluids: From thorax, abdomen, joints, etc.
Swabs: For pus forming and other bacteria. Swab may be taken from eye, ear, throat, vagina, urethra, ulcers, wounds, etc.
Skin scrapings: For *leprae bacilli* or other bacteria.

Specimen Containers

- They should be securely close by screw type caps or well-fitting stoppers.
- They should be properly labeled.
- They should be sterilized if the specimen is to be cultured.

Bacterial Contamination of Specimen

Bacterial contamination of specimens can be prevented generally as described below:

- That cotton-wool plugs or bottle lids removed from cultures are not placed on the bench. They should be properly kept with, between last two fingers. The mouth of tubes or bottles should be sterilized by flaming before the lids are replaced.
- The wireloops, needles, forceps, or scalpel blades are sterilized by flaming before and after being used for inoculating or touching culture media.
- All pipettes should be plugged with non-absorbent cotton-wool and sterilized.
- All petri dishes, tubes, etc., used in preparing culture media are properly washed and sterilized.

Avoiding Infection of Laboratory Workers

- Use of laboratory coat which serves as protection to clothings.
- Washing of hand after handling infected specimen.
- No smoking and eating should be permitted in the working laboratory.
- Any material (infected) accidentally spilt on the bench or in the centrifuge is wiped out with disinfectant on a small piece of cloth which can be discarded into the disinfectant solution.
- All bacterial cultures and infected glasswares after use are discarded into suitable disinfectant containers and autoclaved before washing.

Section 3: Microbiology

- The laboratory benches and equipment such as centrifuge buckets used in the work, are wiped with a disinfectant cloth at the end of each day's work.
- In some cases, the laboratory workers undergo appropriate vaccination, e.g. typhoid, cholera, tuberculosis, etc.

Morphology and Examination of Bacteria

Bacteria are classified by their shape or morphology as under:

Cocci

They are round or oval-shaped bacteria measuring about 0.5 to 1 μ in diameter. They can be of following forms:
- *Diplococci* which are arranged in pairs (**Fig. 4.1A**)
- *Streptococci* which are arranged in chains (**Fig. 4.1B**)
- *Staphylococci* where cocci are arranged in groups or bunches (**Fig. 4.1C**).

Bacilli

- They are rod-like bacteria (**Fig. 4.2A**).
- They range in size from 1 to 10 μ long and 0.3 to 1 μ in thickness.

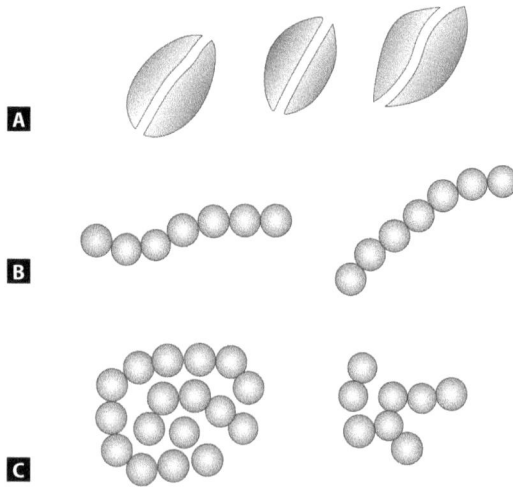

Figs 4.1A to C: Cocci: (A) Diplococci; (B) Streptococci and (C) Staphylococci

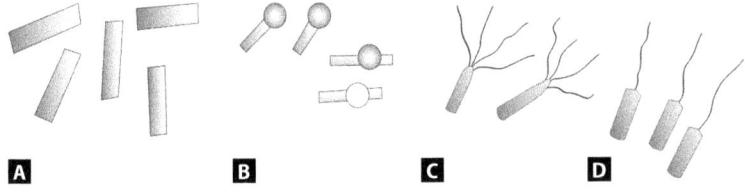

Figs 4.2A to D: Bacilli

- They have their ends rounded or square.
- Some bacilli from spores, when conditions are not favorable for their growth. Spored bacteria are difficult to kill. Some bacilli bear spores towards one end while in other it may be in the middle (**Fig. 4.2B**).
- Many bacteria are motile. They move with the help of a structure called flagella (**Fig. 4.2C**). Flagella may be present at one end of bacilli (**Fig. 4.2D**) or it may be surrounding the entire bacteria.

Bacilli may be of the following shapes:

Vibrio

- Vibrio are small curved like comma, measuring about 3 to 4 μ long and 0.5 μ thick (**Fig. 4.3A**)
- They are very actively motile
- Vibrio has flagellum at one end.

Chinese Letter

Chinese letter arrangement is shown by some bacteria (**Fig. 4.3B**) like *Diphtheria bacilli*.

Spirochetes

Spirochetes (**Fig. 4.3C**) have following features:
- They are thin
- Size may be 5 to 15 μ in length and 0.1 μ in thickness with regular coils
- They can be classified as under:
  - *Treponemae* which are thin spirochetes 5 to 15 μ long by 0.1 μ thick with regular coils.
  - *Borrelia* are large spirochetes about 10 to 30 μ long and 0.5 μ thick with wide irregular coils.

Section 3: Microbiology

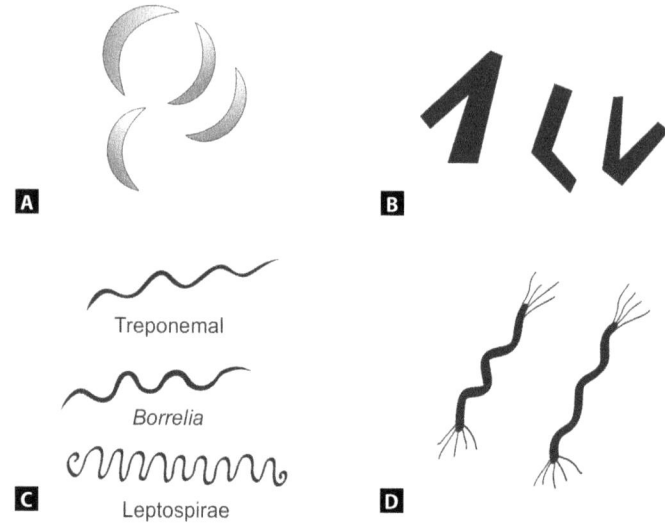

Figs 4.3A to D: Shapes of bacilli: (A) *Vibrio*; (B) Chinese letter; (C) Spirochetes and (D) *Spirilla*

- *Leptospirae* are 5 to 15 μ long and 0.1 μ thick with many small tightly packed coils which are difficult to distinguish. The ends are hooked.

Spirilla

Spirilla are thin, regular, coiled, bacilli about 3 μ to 4 μ long. Each coil measuring 1 μ. They may move by groups of flagella at both ends and not, like the spirochetes, by body movement (**Fig. 4.3D**).

Demonstration of Bacteria in Unstained Preparations

- The easiest and simplest method of studying the bacteria is to examine wet, unstained preparation directly under the microscope.
- Motility, i.e. movement of the bacteria can be seen under the microscope. Hanging-drop preparation is made for this purpose.

Hanging-Drop Preparation

- A clean coverslip is ringed with vaseline or plasticine.
- A drop of bacterial suspension is kept in the middle of coverslip.

- Now a clean glass slide is kept on it carefully, so that coverslip becomes attached to the slide.
- Drop of suspension should not touch either the slide or the ring.
- This preparation is turned so that coverslip is uppermost.
- Study it under the microscope by placing it on microscope stage.
- Focus the edge of drop.
- If the bacteria move actively in different directions, then they are motile.
- If they do not move at all, then they are non-motile.
- Movements because of vibrations of particles result when they struck by surrounding fluid molecules is false motility. It is called Brownian movements.

Demonstration of Bacteria in Stained Preparation

- Staining permits bacteria to be seen more clearly than in direct preparation.
- Staining helps to group the organism
- It helps to identify bacteria roughly.

Some of the important staining methods are:

Methylene Blue

It is a simple method of staining bacteria to show their morphology.

Principle: Methylene blue stains bacteria blue only showing their morphology.

Requirements: Methylene blue ....1 gm
             Distilled water .....200 ml
Dissolve the stain in water and store in bottles

Procedure

- Take a clean slide.
- Spread the specimen like, pus, sputum, etc., on a slide.
- Just warm the slide by passing over the flame once or twice.
- Cover it with methylene blue stain.
- Wait for 3 minutes.
- Wash the smear with water and let the slide stand in a draining rack to dry.

Microscopic Examination

Focus the slide under microscope and use low power than high power and finally oil immersion lenses.

Results

Bacteria are seen as blue-colored structures.

Uses

- We can see the presence or absence of bacteria in smear.
- We can know the shape of rounded bacteria (cocci) or elongated rod-like bacilli.
- We may find out arrangement, i.e. chains of oval or rounded bacteria (cocci), clusters of cocci or pairs of cocci.
- It is possible to demonstrate stain deposits at the ends of bacterial small oval rods. It is called bipolar staining and is found in bacteria causing plague disease.

Gram's Staining

Principle

The basic dye (methyl violet) is retained even after decolorization with acetone in gram-positive bacteria. In gram-negative bacteria on decolorization with acetone, basic dye comes out.

Procedure

- Spread the material containing bacteria on a clean glass slide and dry it.
- Pass the slide over the flame once or twice to fix the smear.
- Cover the smear with crystal violet for 1 minute.
- Wash the slide with water and cover the smear with gram's iodine for 1 minute.
- Drain off gram's iodine.
- Add acetone over the smear and immediately wash the slide with water.
- Cover the smear with diluted carbol fuchsin (1:20). Keep it up for 1 to 2 minutes.
- Wash the slide with water and then dry it and see the smear under microscope (oil immersion).

- Keep the condenser upward.
- Gram-positive bacteria are seen deep violet in color.
- Gram-negative bacteria look pink colored.

Ziehl-Neelsen Staining

Principle

The bacteria which retain carbol fuchsin even after decolorization with acid (20% sulfuric acid) are called acid-fast bacilli, e.g. tubercle bacilli.

Procedure

- Make smear of specimen like sputum by spreading over clean glass slide and dry it.
- Place the slide on two glass rods with the smear facing upwards.
- Cover the smear with strong carbol fuchsin.
- Heat the slide from below till steam starts appearing.
- Wait for 5 to 7 minutes.
- Do not allow the slide to dry of carbol fuchsin.
- Wash the slide with distilled water.
- Add 20% sulfuric acid over the smear and wait for 2½ minutes.
- Wash the smear with water and again keep 20% sulfuric acid for 2½ minutes. Look the smear which would be faint pink in color.
- Add absolute alcohol for 2 minutes, if the specimen is urine.
- Wash it with water.
- Add methylene blue counterstain over smear and keep it for 1 minute.
- Wash the slide with water.
- Dry it and see under the microscope (oil immersion).
- Acid-fast bacilli (e.g. tubercle bacilli) are seen as :
    - Bright red in color
    - Bacilli are straight or curved
    - About 1 to 4 µ
    - May be arranged in group of 3 to 10 bacilli.

Albert Staining

Principle

Metachromatic granules of diphtheria bacilli are stained bluish when treated with a mixture of toluidine blue and malachite green.

Procedure

- Make a smear by spreading the specimen over a clean glass slide.
- Dry the smear and fix it by passing over flame twice or thrice.
- Cover the smear with Albert stain I which contains:

Toluidine blue	1.5 gm
Malachite green	2.0 gm
Glacial acetic acid	10 ml
Alcohol (25%)	90 ml
Distilled water	1000 ml

- Keep this stain up for 5 minutes.
- Wash with water.
- Now cover the slide with Albert stain II which contains:

Iodine	6 gm
Potassium iodide	9 gm
Distilled water	900 ml

- Keep this stain for 2 to 3 minutes
- Wash with water.
- Study it under the microscope using oil immersion objective
- Bacilli are seen as green in color. Metachromatic granules are bluish black.

Sterilization

It is a process of killing all living microorganisms including spores.
It is done using the following methods:

Physical Methods

Physical methods include the following:
- *Heating*:
  - *Dry heat*:
    i. Red heat sterilizes the articles when they are kept in a flame until they become red hot like wireloop, points of forceps, etc.
    ii. Incineration is a method of sterilization by burning, e.g. surgical dressing material, discarded material from clinical laboratories, etc.
    iii. Flaming is used for sterilizing the mouth of tubes, glass slides, etc. The articles are passed through flame without making them red hot.

iv. Hot air oven is used for sterilization of glasswares, oils, etc. Articles are heated in it at 160°C for 1 hour.
   v. Infrared rays.
- *Moist heat*:
   i. Pasteurization is heating at 62°C for 15 to 20 minutes or at 72°C for few seconds. It is used to sterilize milk, etc.
   ii. Inspissation is heating at 75 to 80°C for 1 hour up to 3 days.
   iii. Steamers are used to sterilize the articles like clothes at 100°C for 90 minutes.
   iv. Autoclavation is a method of sterilization at 121°C and pressure 15 lbs for 15 to 20 minutes. It is the best method of sterilization as spores are also killed along with other microorganisms.
- Radiations like gamma rays ultraviolet are used to sterilize plastic articles like disposable syringes.
- Filtration is the method of sterilization where bacteria are caught in small pores of filter and sterilized material passes through, e.g. Earthenware filter (like Berkefeld filter, Chamberland filter), Seitz filter, membrane filter, etc.
- Sunlight.

Chemical Methods
- Ethylene oxide can kill bacteria, viruses and bacterial spores
- Formaldehyde can kill bacteria, viruses and spores
- Glutaraldehyde can also kill bacteria, viruses and spores
- Lysol used at a 2% concentration is used to disinfect glassware, e.g. glass slides and tubes
- Iodine can kill bacteria, viruses and spores
- Alcohol 70% is used to kill bacteria
- Chlorine
- Savlon
- Detergents like soap.

Disinfection of Important Articles
Airways and Endotracheal Tubes
- Single use or autoclaved tubes should be used.
- Disinfection done with 2% glutaraldehyde.

Ampoules

Neck of ampoule is wiped with 70% alcohol and allowed to dry before opening of ampoules.

Bedpans

- Must wear apron and gloves before handling bedpans
- They may be emptied using disposable wooden spatula and paper
- Bedpan can be washed with top phenol for 10 minutes. In case of stools, disinfection with 2% phenol is done for one hour and then it is washed with tap water

Urinals

- Empty the urinals
- Wash with water
- Put urinals in drum of water kept at 80°C for 10 minutes
- Alternatively urinals may be treated with 2% phenol for 15 minutes.

Bedding

- Every week blanket must be changed and used blanket must be sent to laundry.
- Bedsheet should be changed daily or whenever spoiled
- Bedframe should be cleaned with detergent and water after patient is discharged.

Mattresses

- Mattress must be covered with impermeable cover.
- Wipe mattress cover with detergent before bed making.
- Wipe mattress cover with 2% phenol or 5% Savlon or 1% hydrogen peroxide.
- If heavily contaminated then it must be fumigated.
- Pillow should also be treated like mattress as described above.

Blood Spill

- Cover blood spill area with absorbent
- Now pour 1% hypochlorite or 2% carbolic acid

- Leave it for 10 minutes
- Remove with gloves
- Wash the area with disinfectant

Blood Stained Linen

- Soak in fresh bleach solution for 3 minutes.
- Now send linen to laundry.

Bowls

- Bowls should be cleaned with 2% carbolic acid or 5% Lysol or 5% hypochlorite. After rinsing with water it should be kept inverted.
- Surgical bowls may be autoclaved.

Cheatle Forceps

- They may be autoclaved or boiled.
- Forceps may be stored in 2% Savlon.

Thermometers

- Clean the thermometer with 70% alcohol or 2% Savlon. It is done for thermometer that is used auxiliary.
- Clean the thermometer with clean water before use, dry it and then use it. This is done for rectal thermometer

Buckets

- Can be washed and dried.
- They should be kept inverted before use.

Catheter

- Can be discarded after use
- Can be autoclaved

Cytoscope

- It should be kept in 2% glutaraldehyde solution.
- It could be used often by keeping it in glutaraldehyde for 9 to 10 hour.

Endoscope

- It should be kept in 2% glutaraldehyde solution.
- It needs to be treated with glutaraldehyde solution for 10 to 30 minutes in between use.

Culturing of Bacteria

It is useful technique for identification of bacteria. It is also helpful in finding antibacterial substances which can kill the bacteria.

Requirements for Bacterial Food

- Food required for bacteria may be given in the form of media-like peptone water, nutrient broth, etc. Nutrient broth is prepared from meat extract or digested meat. Bacteria with the help of enzymes get their food from nutrient broth in the form of nitrogen, carbon, mineral salts, special growth factors and moisture.
- Temperature required by most of diseases causing bacteria is 37°C.
- Oxygen is necessary for the growth of some bacteria. These bacteria are called aerobes.
- Some bacteria do not require oxygen. As a matter of fact, oxygen is harmful for their growth. Such bacteria are called anaerobes.
- Acid or alkaline nature of a substance is called pH. Usually, bacteria require neutral or slightly alkaline pH (7 to 7.6).
- Some bacteria grow within few hours. There are few bacteria which require several days to grow, e.g. tubercle bacilli.

Culture Media

- Culture media gives artificial conditions which are similar to natural conditions, for the growth of bacteria.
- There are mainly two types of media:
    - Liquid media
    - Solid media

Containers Required for the Preparation of Media

- Flasks plugged with cotton-wool and should be clean and sterilized.
- Test tubes plugged with cotton wool and must be clean and sterilised.
- Screw-capped bottles of different sizes, clean and properly sterilized.
- Petri dishes of different sizes (cleaned and properly sterilized).

Common Ingredients Required for the Preparation of Media

- Distilled water
- Agar-agar which is prepared from a special type of seaweeds. It melts at 95°C and solidifies at 42°C. It is used in the concentration of 1 to 2%
- Peptone is prepared from lean meats like heart. It is water soluble
- Meat extract is prepared by boiling fine meat (lean beef) in water. After removing fat, it is evaporated till dark paste is obtained, it is meat extract
- Yeast extract is prepared from washed cells of yeast
- Blood is usually taken from sheep. Blood may also be taken from rabbit, horse or man
- Serum is obtained from blood of sheep or horse or rabbit.

Liquid Media

Broth

- It is clear straw-colored made from meat extract. It is also called nutrient broth.
- It may be used for the growth of many disease producing bacteria.
- It forms the basis of all culture media.
- It is usually kept in tubes.

Peptone Water

- It is clear water-colored media
- It is kept in tubes
- It is commonly used in bacteriology laboratory
- It forms the basis of all culture media.

Sugar Media

They are prepared by using:

Peptone water 100 ml
Sugar (glucose or lactose or maltose or sucrose) 1 gm
Andrade's indicator 1%
- Distribute into sterilized tubes containing Durham's fermentation tubes kept inverted.
- The sugar media are sterilized by steaming on 3 consecutive days.

Solid Media

Cystine Lactose Electrolyte Deficient (CLED) Medium

- CLED medium is a good differential medium
- It differentiates the lactose fermenting from the non-lactose fermenting organism.

It contains:
Peptic digest animals tissue 4.00 gm
Casein enzyme hydrolysate 4.00 gm
Beef extract 3.00 gm
Lactose 10.0 gm

Method of Preparation

- Dissolve above contents by heating the mixture
- Adjust the pH 7.4 to 7.5
- Sterilize it by autoclaving at 121°C for 15 minutes
- It is poured in petri dishes
- Store in refrigerators

Uses

- Electrolyte deficiency prevents the swarming of protons species
- Organism ferments lactose and produce acid which turn the bromothymol blue to yellow and colonies appear yellow.

Nutrient Agar

It consists of:
- Agar 2 gm
- Peptone water 100 ml
- Sodium chloride 0.5 gm
  - Heat the contents at 100°C and mix well
  - Sterilization is done by autoclaving

- It is put in Petri dishes
- It is light yellow-colored media.

Blood Agar

It consists of:
- Sheep blood 7 to 10 ml
- Nutrient agar 100 ml
    - Blood 10 ml is added to melted nutrient agar at 45°C
    - After mixing it well, put it into Petri dish
    - It is bright red in color.

Chocolate Agar

- It is also called heated blood agar medium.
- It is prepared by heating blood agar medium at 80°C until it turns brown.

MacConkey's Medium

- It contains:

Agar	10 gm
Bile salt	5 gm
Peptone	20 gm
Sodium chloride	5 gm
Water	1000 ml

- Dissolve above contents by heating the mixture
- Add lactose 20 gm and adjust pH 7.4 to 7.5.
- Add 10 ml ot 1% aqueous neutral red.
- Sterilize it by autoclaving at 107°C for 10 minutes.
- It is poured in Petri dishes and stored in refrigerator.
- It is brown-colored medium.

Loeffler Serum Slope

- Take 75 ml horse serum.
- Add 25 ml dextrose broth
- Dispense in sterilized MacConkey bottles.
- Put the bottles containing media in a slanting position in an inspissator or water bath.
- Keep the temperature 75 to 80°C for 1 hour and repeat it for 3 days.
- Medium in bottle is pale white in color.

Löwenstein-Jensen Medium (in Slope)

- It consists of:

Potassium dihydrogen phosphate (KH_2PO_4)	4 gm
Magnesium sulfate anhydrous ($MgSO_4.7H_2O$)	0.4 gm
Magnesium citrate	1.0 gm
Asparagine	6.0 gm
Glycerol	20 ml
Distilled water	1000 ml

- Dissolve these and steam for 2 hours.
- Clean fresh egg and break open into a sterilized graduate cylinder. Take 1600 ml of egg fluid, filter it and mix with above-mentioned mixture.
- Add 50 ml of 1% malachite green.
- Put it in sterilized MacConkey's bottles properly closed with screw cap.
- Keep these bottle in a inspissator for 1 hour.
- Repeat it for three days.
- Store this media in refrigerator at 7.5.
- This media is used for the growth of tubercle bacilli.

Robertson's Cooked Meat Media (RCM)

- It contains:
  - Minced beef heart 500 gm
  - Sodium hydroxide (N/20) = 500 ml
- Cook the contents for 20 minutes.
- Filter through gauze (3 layers) and squeeze.
- Dry the meat particles at 80°C for 15 to 20 minutes by spreading over a filter paper.
- Distribute meat in MacConkey's bottles (or tubes (5° x (5°)/(8°)) making a layer of 1 inch.
- Add 10 ml nutrient broth in each tube.
- Sterilize by autoclaving at 121°C for 20 minutes.
- Adjust the pH after sterilization at 7.5
- This media is used for:
  - Growing anaerobic bacteria
  - Stock culture (preservation).

Culture Methods

Following points must be remembered about culture methods:
- Check the number of specimen.
- Keep all the items which are required for culturing, ready.
- Do not talk while working.
- Always work around spirit lamp with fans off.
- As a routine use both enriched media (blood agar, chocolate agar) and selective media (MacConkey's media, DCA media).

Procedure
- First of all dry Petri dishes containing media in an incubator.
- Take a wireloop (platinum which is 2½" long wire with loop at its end about 2 mm in diameter (**Figs 4.4A to E**).
- Sterilize the loop by placing it over spirit lamp flame till it becomes red hot.
- Cool it and dip it in the clinical specimen which may contain bacteria.
- Place the material on the surface of solid media, i.e. blood agar towards edge (primary inoculum).

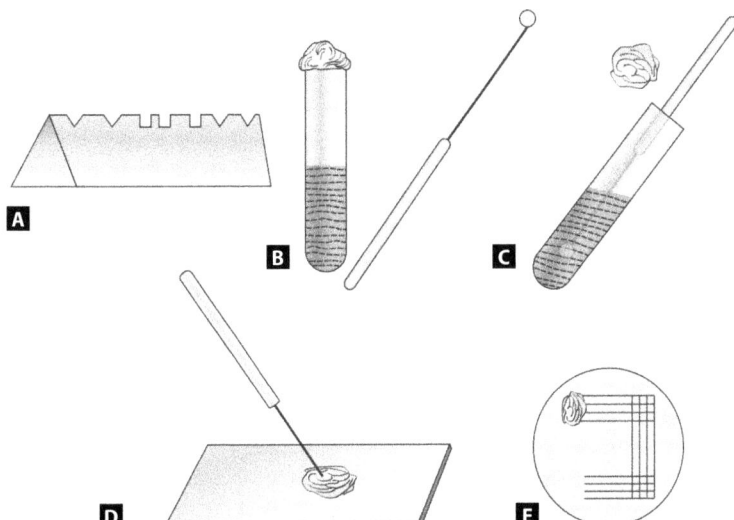

Figs 4.4A to E: (A) Stand for wireloop; (B) Wireloop; (C) Touching the wireloop with bacterial growth; (D) Preparation of smear on glass slide; (E) Spreading

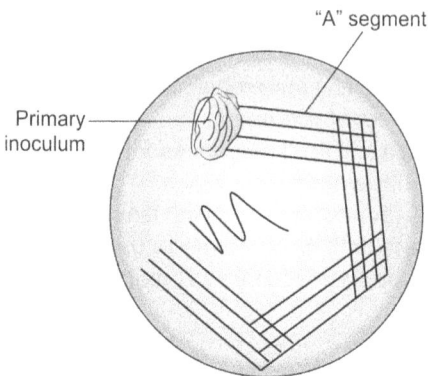

Fig. 4.5: Bacterial growth

- This material is spread thinly over the surface of blood agar medium plate in series of parallel lines in different sections of the plate.
- Like this spread, the material on MacConkey's agar medium.
- Invert plates and keep in an incubator at 37°C overnight.
- After incubation study, the plates (blood agar and MacConkey). We may find clumps of colonies (confluent growth) at the site of primary inoculum. Well-separated colonies are present over last few streaks (**Figs 4.4 and 4.5**).

Biochemical Test

Catalase Test

- Mix a colony in 1 ml of 1% solution of Tween 80 in a screw-cap bottle.
- Add to it 0.5 ml of 20 vol hydrogen peroxide and replace cap of bottle.
- Appearance of bubbles or effervescence indicates presence of catalase (test positive).

Coagulase Test

Slide Method

Mix a colony in 1 ml of 1% solution of Tween 80 in a screw cap bottle.
- If no clumps appear dip straight wire in rabbit plasma and stir the mixture with straight wire.
- In positive test, clumps appear with 10 seconds.

Test Tube Test

- Add 0.2 ml plasma to 0.8 ml of nutrient broth in a test tube.
- Add 0.1 ml of overnight growth in broth
- Incubate at 37° C in water bath for 6 hours.
- Examine the tube after every 2 hours for formation of clots.
- In positive test, clot formation is positive.

Hydrogen Sulfide Test

- Dip a strip of filter paper with 10% solution a basic lead acetate and dry it.
- Place this strip in top of nutrient broth tube containing colonies of bacteria.
- Incubate the tube at 37°C overnight.
- Blackening of paper means production of hydrogen sulfide and test is positive.

Indole Test

- Take peptone water containing bacterial colonies incubated at 37°C for few days.
- Add few drops of Kovac's reagent.
- A pink-colored ring formation means test is positive.

Kovac's reagent is prepared by mixing the following:
- P-dimethyl-aminobenzaldehyde—5 gm
- Add to ↓
- Mixture of amyl alcohol (75 ml) + concentrated sulfuric acid (25 ml).

Methyl Red Test

- Add a colony of bacteria in a test tube containing glucose phosphate broth.
- Incubate it at 37°C for few days.
- Add a few drops of methyl red solution.
- Red coloration means test is positive.
  Methyl red solution is prepared as under:

Methyl red	0.1 gm
Ethanol	300 ml
Distilled water	200 ml

Nitrate Reduction Test

- Colony is mixed in nitrate broth (containing 1% potassium nitrate).
- Incubate at 37°C for 5 days.
- Add 1 to 2 drops of a mixture of sulfanilic acid and naphthylamine (mixed in equal quantity).
- Appearance of red color means test is positive.

Oxidase Test

- Soak piece of filter paper in 1% aqueous tetramethyl p-phenylene-diamine dihydrochloride.
- Scrap young bacterial colony with a clean and sterilized platinum loop (over flame of spirit lamp)
- Rub it on soaked filter paper piece.
- Appearance of deep blue or deep purple color within 10 seconds means oxidase test is positive.

Phenylalanine Test (PPA)

- Take phenylalanine medium slope.
- Apply the dense growth over this slope.
- Incubate at 37°C for overnight
- After incubation add few drops of 10% aqueous ferric chloride solution.
- Appearance of green color means test is positive.

Triple Sugar Iron (TSI)

- Take straight wire properly sterilized and dip in growth of bacteria.
- Stab the medium in test tube with this straight wire charged with bacterial growth, into butt and slant.
- Incubate it at 37°C.
- Blackening means production of hydrogen sulfide, yellow discoloration means fermentation of sugars. Breaking or cracks of medium means gas formation.

Christensen's Urease Medium Test

- Take a container containing medium in slope form.
- Apply bacterial growth heavily on the slope.

- Incubate at 37°C for overnight.
- Appearance of red color mean test is positive.

Voges-Proskauer Test
- Colony of bacteria is mixed in glucose phosphate medium and incubate at 37°C for 48 hours.
- Add 1 ml of 40% potassium hydroxide and 3 ml of 5% α-naphthol in absolute alcohol.
- Development of pink color in 2 to 5 minutes changing into crimson in 30 minutes means test is positive.

Brief Description of Some Bacteria

Staphylococcus aureus
Morphology: Gram-positive cocci (1 micron) arranged in clusters.

Culture: On blood agar plate, colonies grow as:
- Smooth
- Circular
- Pinhead size
- Golden yellow colored
- Showing complete (beta) hemolysis around colonies

Motility: Non-motile (hanging-drop preparation)

Biochemical test
- Catalase test—positive
- Coagulase test—positive

Diseases: Pus formation, pneumonia, wound infection, skin boils, etc.

Streptococcus pyogenes
Morphology: Gram-positive cocci arranged in chains

Culture: On blood agar, medium colonies are:
- Pin point
- Complete hemolysis (β-hemolysis) around colonies

Motility: Non-motile (hanging drop preparation)
Biochemical test
- Catalase test—negative

Disease: Rheumatic fever

Pneumococci

Morphology: They are gram-positive cocci arranged in pairs. They are capsulated.

Culture: On blood agar, plate colonies are seen as:
- Small in size and after sometime show depressed center and raised margins (draughtsman colonies).
- Zone of hemolysis around colony is green (α-hemolysis).

Motility: Non-motile (hanging drop preparation)

Biochemical test:
- Bile solubility test—positive
- Optochin sensitivity test—positive
- Inulin fermentation—positive

Diseases: Pneumonia, meningitis, etc.

Gonococci

Morphology: They are gram-negative cocci (bean or kidney-shaped) arranged in pairs.

Culture: On chocolate (heated blood-blood agar), colonies are seen as:
- Small
- Round
- Raised
- Smooth

Motility: Non-motile (hanging-drop preparation).

Biochemical reactions:
- Oxidase test—positive
- Fermentation of glucose without gas formation is positive.

Disease: Gonorrhea

Clostridium tetani

Morphology:
- They are gram-positive bacilli
- They show terminal spherical spores (drum-stick appearance)

Culture: On blood agar (without oxygen in the environment) shows following feature:

From primary inoculum, the growth spreads all over as a mass of fine filaments.

Motility: Motile bacilli

Biochemical tests:
- Robertson cooked meat media shown black coloration due to proteolytic action of *Clostridium tetani*.
- No sugar fermentation

Disease: Tetanus

Tubercle Bacilli (*Mycobacterium tuberculosis*)
- They are both acid-fast and alcohol fast
- They are rod-shaped or slightly curved and in beaded forms

Culture: Colonies appear on Löwenstein-Jensen slope (green colored) with features as under:
- Pigmented, usually yellowish colored growth
- They are not easy to emulsify in normal saline solution

Motility: Non-motile

Disease: Tuberculosis

Diphtheria Bacilli

Morphology:
- They are gram-positive bacilli
- They are arranged in Chinese letters
- Metachromatic granules are seen in Albert-stained smear as bluish-black granules.

Culture

- On blood agar, Loeffler's serum slope and blood tellurite medium. *Diphtheria bacilli* are grown.
- On Loeffler's serum slope, colonies are small and circular which become thick with irregular borders.

- On blood tellurite medium, colonies are gray to white in color and 2 to 4 mm in size.
- On blood agar, colonies are small and may be hemolytic.

Motility: Non-motile bacilli

Biochemical tests: Sugar fermentation (of glucose and maltose) is there and with formation of acid only.

Diseases: They cause disease known as diphtheria due to the production of powerful toxin.

Salmonella typhi

Morphology: They are gram-negative bacilli.

Culture: On MacConkey agar medium, colonies are:
- Colorless
- Large in size 2 to 4 mm
- Mucoid
- Circular

Motility: Motile

Biochemical tests:
    Indole test—negative
    Methyl red test—positive
    Voges-Proskauer—negative
    Hydrogen sulfide—positive
    Citrate test—positive
    Urease test—negative
    Fermentation of glucose-positive with only acid production.

Disease: Typhoid fever.

Vibrio Cholerae (Cholera Bacilli)

Vibrio Cholera

Morphology: It is gram-negative bacilli. It is slightly curved and comma shaped.

Culture: On MacConkey agar medium, colonies are:
- Colorless
- Moist
- 1 to 2 mm in size

Biochemical tests:
- Oxidase test—positive
- Indole test—positive
- Nitrate reduction test—positive
- Glucose fermentation—only acid production
- Sucrose fermentation—only acid production
- Mannitol fermentation—only acid production

Disease: Cholera

Treponema pallidum

Morphology: It is about 10 µ in length and 0.1 µ in thickness and it consists of 6 to 12 small regular coils.

Culture: It cannot be cultured.

Biochemical test: Not useful.

Disease: Syphilis.

Bacteriological Examination of Water

Collection of Water

- Samples of water are collected in a suitable sterilized glass bottle with stopper or cap.
- About 250 ml of water should be collected.
- If water sample is chlorinated, sodium thiosulfate should be added to water sample.
- To collect the water from tap, clean the tap with a piece of clean cloth. Heat the tap with flames of spirit lamp. Open the tap and allow to flow the water from tap for 1 to 2 minutes. Take sterilized bottle and fill it with water. Replace the stopper. Dispatch it. Along with bottle send required information like date and time of collection, name of place, etc.
- Water sample can also be collected from wells, pond, river, springs, etc.

Packing and Dispatching of Water Sample

- Bottles should be despatched in a strong box to prevent breakage.
- Bottles should be kept cool by placing ice cubes between bottles.
- Bottles should reach the laboratory within 6 hours of collection.

Section 3: Microbiology

Procedure for Bacteriological Examination of Drinking Water
- Incubate the above tubes at 37°C for 24 hours.
- Identify the tubes showing acid production and gas formation.
- Now consult McCrady table and find out presumed coliform count (**Fig. 4.6**).

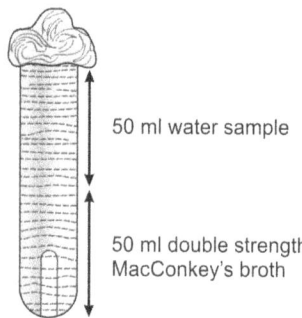

50 ml water sample

50 ml double strength MacConkey's broth

One test tube with capacity of more than 100 ml

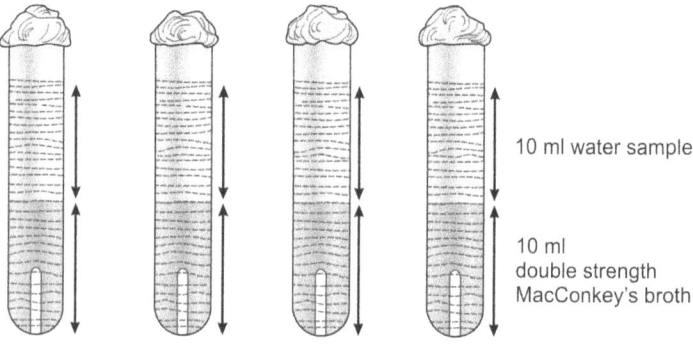

10 ml water sample

10 ml double strength MacConkey's broth

5 test tubes each with capacity of over 20 ml

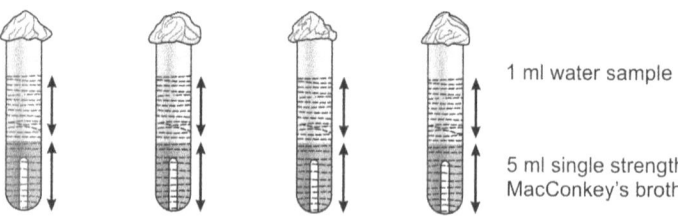

1 ml water sample

5 ml single strength MacConkey's broth

Fig. 4.6: Bacteriological examination of water

MYCOLOGY

It is the branch of medical microbiology which deals with the study of fungi. Fungi occurs mainly in three forms:
1. Yeast form
2. Hyphae form which are thread-like structure. It may be divided into parts by septa (aseptate hyphae). It may be without septa (aseptate hyphae)
3. Mycelium is a group of hyphase.

Classification

Diseases causing fungi (**Fig. 4.7**) are classified as under:
- Superficial fungi causing diseases of skin, hair, nails, e.g. dermatophytes.
- Subcutaneous fungi cause infection of structures just below the skin, e.g. *Candida, Rhinosporidium seeberi*, etc.
- Systemic fungi cause infection of many organs like lungs, brain, etc., e.g. *Cryptococcus, Histoplasma*, etc.

Methods for Studying Fungi in Specimen

Collection of Specimen
- Skin scrap, nails and hair clipping are collected into a piece of clean tissue paper.
- Fold this paper properly and send it to laboratory.
- Sputum, pus, spinal fluid and biopsy of tissues are collected in sterilized container.

Microscopic Examination
- Sputum, pus, biopsy are placed in 10% KOH drop on a clean glass cover.
- Skin scrap, nail clips and hair clips placed into a clean glass slide.
- Add 10% potassium hydroxide solution drop.
- Cover it with coverslip and seal the margin of coverslip with nail polish.
- Keep it in an incubator till material is dissolved.
- Examine under microscope to find fungi (yeast, budding yeasts or hyphae).
- Dried smear is fixed and then Gram's staining is done.

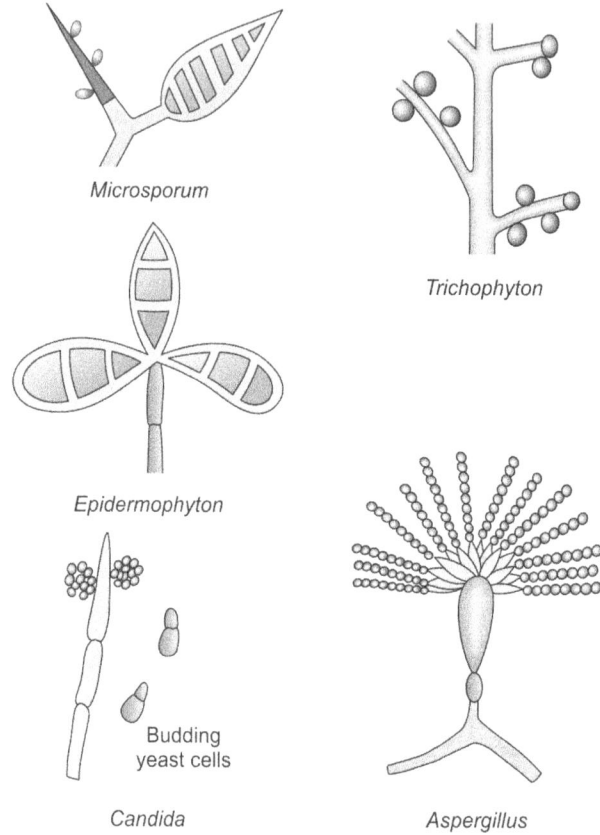

Fig. 4.7: Fungal organisms causing diseases in man

Cultural Examination

- The scrapping of skin, nail or hairclips, biopsy material, sputum, etc. are placed on Sabouraud's dextrose agar medium (two tubes per specimen).
- Incubate one tube at 37°C and the other one at room temperature (22°C).
- Incubation is done for 3 weeks.
- As soon as growth appears, mix the growth gently in a drop of lactophenol cotton blue kept on a clean glass slide.
- Cover it with coverslip and study under microscope for hyphae and yeast cells, etc.

Chapter 4: Microbiology

PARASITOLOGY

It is the branch of science of microbiology dealing with study of parasites which live in man causing diseases. Parasite may be single-celled structure called protozoa and many-celled structure called helminths.

Protozoa

Important protozoa are described as:

Entamoeba histolytica
It is found all over the world and cause dysentery and pus in liver, lungs, brain, etc. It enters the man because of taking food containing cyst form of parasite. In laboratory, it is recognized by studying stool preparation under microscope. It is found in following two forms:
1. Trophozoites
2. Cyst

Trophozoites

- Size 20 to 30 micron (**Fig. 4.8A**)
- Move actively
- Defined into ectoplasma and endoplasma
- Nucleus is centrally placed and nucleolus is also placed in center.
- Cytoplasm contains red blood cells, tissue debris, etc.

Cyst

- Size 6 to 15 micron (**Fig. 4.8B**)
- It has maximum 4 nuclei
- Chromidial bars may be seen in early stages.
- Glycogen mass may be seen in early stages only.

Entamoeba Coli
It is not harmful. It is found in both cystic and trophozoitic forms.

Trophozoites

- Size 20 to 40 micron (**Fig. 4.9A**)
- Sluggishly motile

Section 3: Microbiology

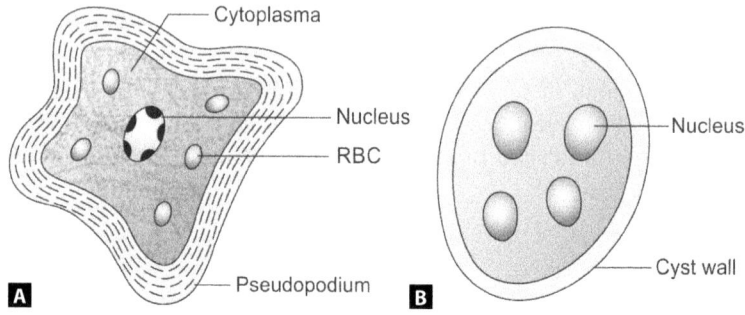

Figs 4.8A and B: (A) Trophozoites; (B) Cyst

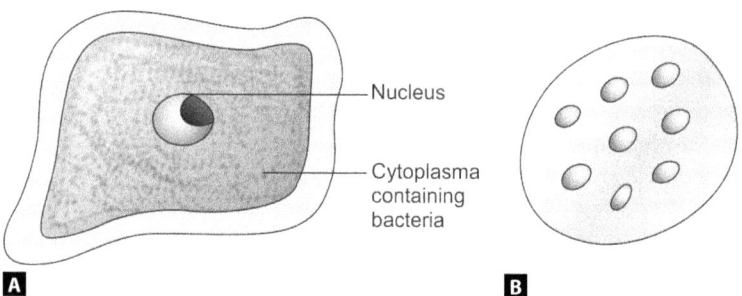

Figs 4.9A and B: (A) Trophozoites; (B) Cyst

- Ectoplasm and endoplasm are not defined
- Cytoplasm contains bacteria only
- Nucleus is present with nucleolous on one side.

Cyst

- Size 15 to 20 micron (**Fig. 4.9B**).
- May have nuclei, 8 in number.
- Glycogen is present in mature cyst (late stages).
- Chromidial bars are thread like.

Giardia lamblia

It occurs in cyst and trophozoite forms. It may produce diarrhea, gas, loss of appetite, abdominal pain, etc.

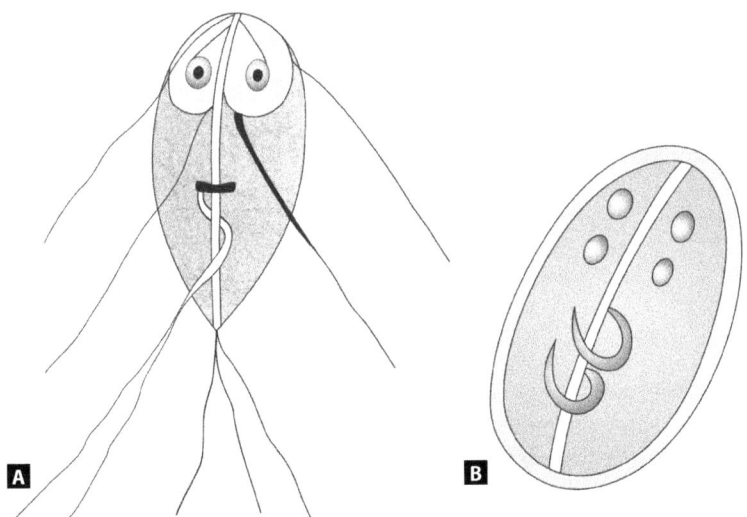

Figs 4.10A and B: (A) Trophozoite; (B) Cyst

Trophozoites

- It is 14 micron long and 7 micron broad (**Fig. 4.10A**)
- Two axostyles
- Two nuclei
- Four pairs of flagella

Cyst

- Size 7 μ broad and 14 μ long (**Fig. 4.10B**)
- Oval in shape
- Four nuclei

Malarial Parasites

There are four species:
1. *Plasmodium vivax*
2. *Plasmodium falciparum*
3. *Plasmodium malariae*
4. *Plasmodium ovale*

They cause disease called malaria in which patient shivers, then feels hot and finally sweating.

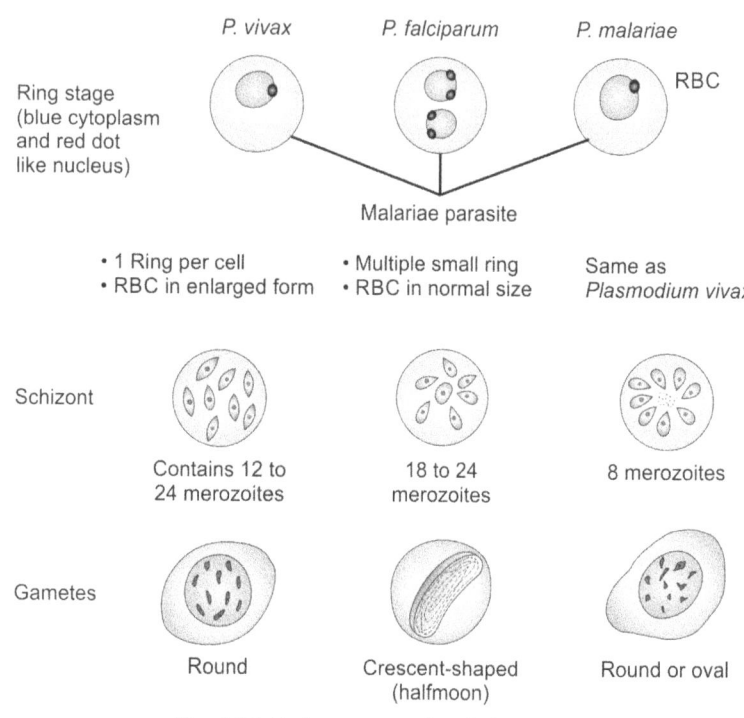

Fig. 4.11: Various stages of malaria parasite

It is found in various forms and are detected in thin and thick blood smear stained with Leishman's stain. Nuclear material is seen pink in color while cytoplasm of material parasite is blue in color (**Fig. 4.11**).

Helminths

Some of the important helminths are discussed here:

Hookworms (*Ancylostoma duodenale*)

- It is responsible for anemia, bronchopneumonia and sometimes dermatitis.
- It enters the body by penetrating the skin between toes of feet.
- It may be found in the forms of eggs and adult worm (**Fig. 4.12**).

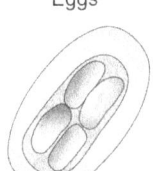

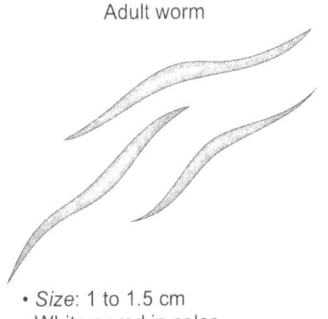

- *Size*: 1 to 1.5 cm
- White or red in color
- Look like a piece of thread

- Oval or rounded
- 30 to 60 micron in size
- Covered by very thin layer shell
- Usually contains 4 gray granular cells (blastomeres)

Fig. 4.12: Hookworm and eggs

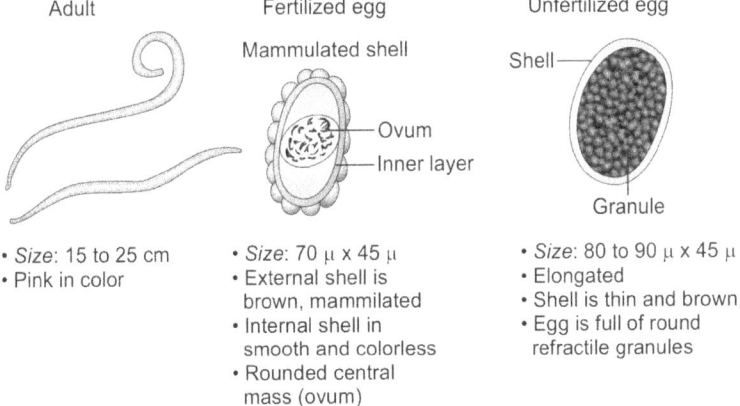

- *Size*: 15 to 25 cm
- Pink in color

- *Size*: 70 μ x 45 μ
- External shell is brown, mammilated
- Internal shell in smooth and colorless
- Rounded central mass (ovum)

- *Size*: 80 to 90 μ x 45 μ
- Elongated
- Shell is thin and brown
- Egg is full of round refractile granules

Fig. 4.13: Roundworms and eggs

Roundworm (*Ascaris lumbricoides*)

- Responsible for malnutrition, intestinal obstruction, cough and fever (in children).
- It enters body by taking food or water containing eggs.
- It is found in adult form and eggs (fertilized and unfertilized) (**Fig. 4.13**)

Pinworm (*Enterobius vermicularis*)

- It is also called seatworm.
- It is responsible for severe itching around anus.

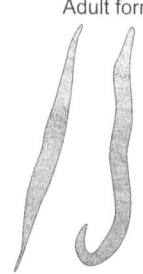 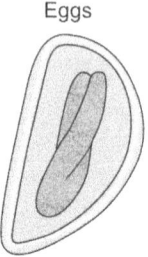

Adult form

- White in color
- *Size*: 0.5 to 1 cm
- Found in stools, around anus and underneath the nails used for scratching the itching part

Eggs

- Colorless
- *Size*: 50 to 60 μ × 30 μ
- Oval with on side convex and other flattened
- Shell in thin
- Usually contains curled up larva

Fig. 4.14: Pinworms and egg

- It enters the body by using hands containing eggs, during eating or drinking.
- It is found in adult form and egg/ova form (**Fig. 4.14**).

Whipworm (*Trichuris trichiura*)

- It is responsible for abdominal pain, appendicitis, mucus and blood-streaked stools and prolapse of rectum.
- It enters the body by eating and drinking things containing eggs of whipworm.
- Eggs finding in stool examination confirms infections with whipworm (**Fig. 4.15**).

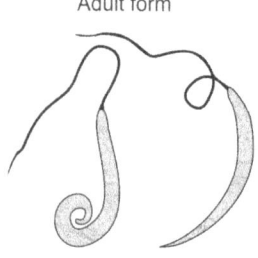 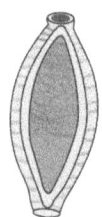

Adult form

- *Size*: 3 to 5 cm in length
- It is whip-like in shape

Eggs

- *Size*: 50 μ × 25 μ
- Barrel shaped
- Shell in thick with two layers
- Rounded colorless plugs at both ends
- Contains granular ovum

Fig. 4.15: Whipworms and egg

Adult form	Eggs
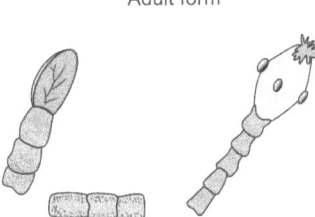	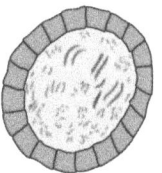
• White or pale blue in color • Total length of worm is 3 to 10 meters • Usually segments are seen • Mature segment in 1 to 3 cm • Segments are studied by gently pressing between 2 slides for arrangement of pores, uterine branches and head (scolex)	• Spherical in shape • Brown in color • Embryophore is radially striated • Oncosphere contains three pairs of hookless

Fig. 4.16: Tapeworm and egg

Tapeworm (*Taenia*)

- It may be beef tapeworm (*Taenia saginata*), pork tapeworm (*Taenia solium*)
- It enters the man by eating raw meat containing larvae (pork or beef)
- Tapeworm is of many meters long lying inside intestine of man.
- Infection with this worm is by studying segments passed by patient along with stools.
- It occurs in adult form and eggs (**Fig. 4.16**).

Dwarf Tapeworm (*Hymenolepis nana*)

- It is found in small intestine
- It enters the man through food or drink containing eggs of this worm
- It may be responsible for pain of abdomen and diarrhea
- It is found in adult form and egg form (**Fig. 4.17**).

IMMUNOLOGY

In the laboratory, generally techniques are based on the following antigen-antibody reactions:
- *Agglutination reactions*: These occur when particulate antigen reacts with antibody in the presence of electrolytes at suitable temperature and pH, e.g. Widal test, C-reactive protein (CRP) test, rheumatoid factor.

Section 3: Microbiology

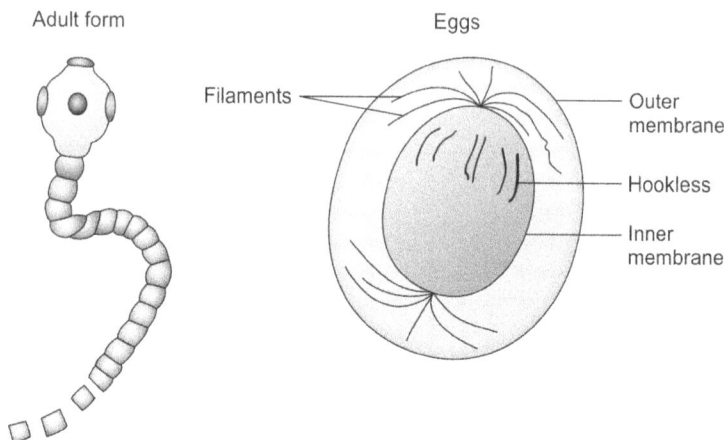

- *Size*: Small (1 to 4 cm) and 1 mm
- Thread like
- It has head (scolex), segments
- Terminal segment separates from dwarf tapeworm
- Spherical or oval
- *Size*: 30 to 45 μ
- Outer membrane thin and colorless
- Oncosphere contains three pairs hookless
- The space between two layers contains yolk granules and polar filament

Fig. 4.17: Dwarf tapeworm and egg

- *Precipitation reactions*: These occur when soluble antigen reacts with antibody in the presence of electrolytes at suitable temperature and pressure, e.g. VDRL test, Kahn's test, etc.
- *Neutralization reactions*: Where antibodies neutralize the effect of antigen, e.g. antistreptolysin O (ASO) test.

Widal Test

Principle
It is an agglutination test and it is done to diagnose typhoid fever.

Requirements
- Widal rack with 4 rows each containing 6 tubes (3 × 3/8")
- Pipettes
- Glass beaker
- Normal saline
- Antigens
  - *S. typhi O* (TO)
  - *S. typhi H* (TH)

- *Flagellar S. paratyphi A* (AH)
- *Flagellar S. paratyphi B* (BH)
- Water bath
- Hand lens/mirror

Procedure

- For each serum sample arrange 4 rows of 6 tubes each in a Widal rack
- Take 5 tubes in another rack for preparing master dilution as under:
  - Take 2.5 ml of normal saline in tube number 1 and 2.5 ml of normal saline in other 4 tubes
  - Add 0.5 ml of test serum in tube number 1 and mix well
  - Take 2.5 ml from tube 1 to tube 2 and mix well. Do it till the last tube
- Transfer 0.5 ml from master dilution to each of corresponding vertical row in test tube
- Place 0.5 ml of normal saline in each tube in 6th row vertically to serve as control
- Add 0.5 ml of TO antigen to each of 6 tubes in the first horizontal row
- Add 0.5 ml of TH antigen to each of 6 tubes in the second horizontal row
- Add 0.5 ml of AH antigen to each of 6 tubes in the third horizontal row
- Add 0.5 ml of BH antigen to each of 6 tubes in the fourth horizontal row
- Now we have dilutions as 1:20, 1:40, 1:80, 1:160, 1:320.
- Shake the rack well to mix and incubate at 37°C overnight.
- Note the agglutination in tubes with the help of hand lens or mirror.
- Reporting is done as under:

	1/20	1/40	1/80	1/160	1/320
TO	+	+	+	+	+
TH	+	+	+	+	+
AH	−	−	−	−	−
BH	+	−	−	−	−

Latex Fixation Test for Rheumatoid Factor

Principle

It is based on principle of clumping or agglutination.

Requirements

- Glass beakers
- Pipettes
- Latex rheumatoid reagent
- Normal saline
- Patient serum
- Positive serum control
- Negative serum control
- Dark slide
- Stirring rods

Procedure

- Dilute patient serum 1:5 (1 part serum + 4 part normal saline)
- Place 1 drop of this diluted serum of the patient and 1 drop each of positive control serum and negative drop serum to different zones on dark slide.
- Add one drop of latex rheumatoid reagent to serum of the patient, and one drop each to positive control and negative control.
- Mix well with stirring rod (one rod for each sample)
- Clumping or agglutination, if appears within 2 minutes, it means test is positive.

C-Reactive Protein (CRP)

Principle

This test is based on agglutination reaction.

Requirements

- Latex CRP reagent consisting of polystyrene particles sensitized with gamma-globulin fraction from specific anti-CRP serum.
- Normal saline
- CRP-positive control
- CRP-negative control
- Graduated pipettes
- Glass beakers
- Dark slide
- Patient serum

Procedure
- Bring serum sample and reagents to room temperature.
- Dilute serum 1:5 (1 part serum + 4 parts normal saline).
- Place one drop of diluted patient serum on test place (dark plate slide).
- Also place 1 drop of positive control serum and drop of negative control serum separately on dark slide.
- Add one drop of CRP reagent (antigen) each to patient serum, positive control serum and negative control serum.
- Mix well with wooden/plastic stick and look for agglutination.
- Clumping or agglutination in patient serum drop means test is positive.

Latex ASO (Antistreptolysin-O)
Principle
Latex ASO test is based on clumping or agglutination.

Requirements
- Beakers
- Pipettes
- Normal saline
- Latex antistreptolysin reagent consisting of suspension of polystyrene latex particles sensitized with streptolysin-O
- Negative control
- Positive control
- Dark slide

Procedure
- Take 5 tubes for one serum sample for ASO test.
- Dilute serum as under:
  Tube I   1:5   (1 part serum + 4 part normal saline)
  Tube II   1:10   (0.5 ml serum from tube I + 0.5 ml normal saline)
  Tube III 1:20   (0.5 ml of serum from tube II + 0.5 ml of normal saline)
  Tube IV   1:30   (1 drop of serum + 29 drops of normal saline)
  Tube V   1:40   (1 drop of serum + 39 drops of normal saline)
- Place one drop of each of the 5 dilution on dark plate
- Also place one drop of positive control serum and one drop of negative control serum on the same dark plate

- Shake the antistreptolysin reagent bottle and transfer one drop each to 5 dilution and two controls
- Stirrer each of them with stirring rods and record the clumping within 2 minutes.

Pregnancy Test (Gravindex Test)

Principle
This test is based on clumping or agglutination.

Requirements
- Dark slide
- Gravindex antiserum (bottle)
- Gravindex antigen (bottle)

Procedure
- Take one drop of Gravindex anti-serum on a clean dark slide
- Add a drop of urine of lady patient
- Mix slowly for 30 seconds by tilting the slide gently
- Now add 2 drops of Gravindex antigen
- Mix gently by tilting the slide slowly
- See if clumping is present within 2 minutes
- No clumping means : Pregnancy—positive
  clumping means: Pregnancy—negative
- Do not forget to test positive and negative control.

Venereal Disease Research Laboratory (VDRL) Test

Principle
It is a precipitation test where antigen (in soluble form) react with antibodies in the presence of electrolytes at neutral pH and at 37°C.

Requirements
- VDRL antigen
- VDRL buffer
- Serum of patient

- 1 ml syringe with 21 gauge needle delivering 60 drops per ml
- Concavity slides measuring 16 mm in diameter and 1.75 mm in depth
- Thirty ml round glass stoppered bottle with narrow mouth and flat bottom
- Pipettes
- Tubes
- Stop watch
- Water bath
- Thermometer.

Procedure

- Pipette 0.4 ml of buffered saline to a bottom of 30 ml round glass stoppered bottle
- Add 0.5 ml of antigen onto the buffered saline within 6 seconds. Rotate the bottle continuously and gently for about 10 seconds
- Add 4.1 ml of buffered saline
- Place the stopper on the bottle mouth and shake bottle from bottom to the top and back for about 30 times within 10 seconds
- Inactivate the serum sample of patient by keeping it at 56°C for 30 minutes in water bath
- Place 0.05 ml of inactivated serum into one concavity of slide
- Also place positive and negative control
- Add one drop (1/60th part of 1 ml) of antigen freshly prepared each onto the serum, positive control and negative control with especially prepared syringe
- Rotate the slide by hand circumscribing a 2 inches diameter circle at 120 times per minute for 4 minutes
- Now look for flocculation with naked eye and microscopically with low power objective
- Appearance of floccules means test is positive. Now dilute the serum 1:2, 1:4, 1:8, 1:16, 1:32, ... and repeat the test to find out titer up to which floccules appear
- Test is positive in patient having syphilis disease.

Kahn's Test

Principle

It is based on a precipitation (antigen is used in solution form).

Requirements

- Kahn's antigen
- Normal saline
- Patient serum
- Kahn's tube rack
- Kahn's pipettes (to measure 0.0125 ml, 0.025 ml and 0.05 ml)
- Pipette to measure 0.15 ml
- Water bath
- Kahn's oscillator
- Buffer
- Hand lens

Procedure

- Mix 1 ml of Kahn's antigen to 1.2 ml of normal saline and mix thoroughly.
- The diluted antigen is allowed to stand at room temperature for 10 minutes.
- Serum of the patient is inactivated by placing the tube (patient serum) in water bath at 56°C for 30 minutes.
- Take 4 test tubes and proceed as under:

	Tube 1	Tube 2	Tube 3	Tube 4
Antigen (freshly diluted)	0.15 ml	0.025 ml	0.0125	0.05
Serum of patient	0.15 ml	0.15 ml	0.15 ml	nil

- Now shake the rack with tubes on Kahn's oscillator (20 oscillation per minute) for 3 minutes.

Normal saline 1.0 ml, 0.5 ml, 0.5 ml, 1 ml.
Now shake the rack containing tube to mix and look for floccules.
- Appearance of floccules means test is positive.
- Test is positive in person suffering from disease syphilis.

ELISA Test

ELISA means enzyme-linked immunosorbent assay. It may be used as diagnostic test as well as epidemiological test for microbial diseases. This test may be done for detection of antibody or antigen. Hormonal assay is also possible with this method. Mainly, ELISA is of two types:
- Sandwich ELISA
- Indirect ELISA

Sandwich ELISA

This technique is used for detection of antigen in the specimen. It is done as under:
- The wells of microtiter plate are coated with antibody against the antigen to be detected
- Test sample is added in coated well
- If antigen is present in test sample, it will bind to coated antibody
- Now antibody coated with conjugate and enzyme is added
- This conjugated antibody attaches to antigen already combined to coated antibody
- Now substrate is added
- In case, there is binding of conjugated antibody to antigen-antibody complex, enzyme will react with substrate to produce color. It happens, if test is positive
- The intensity of color is measured by ELISA reader
- Along with test, positive and negative controls must also be run and tested.
- Incubation and washing is a must to get rid of unbound reagents at every step of this test.

Indirect ELISA

This technique is done to detect antibody from test sample. It is done as:
- The well of microliter plate is coated with antigen
- Test sample is added to coated well
- If antibody is present in test sample, it gets attached to coated antigen
- Now a goat antihuman immunoglobulin antibody conjugated with enzyme is added. It gets attached to antibody
- Now substrate is added. In case, test is positive enzyme acts on substrate to produce color which can be measured using ELISA reader
- Along with the test, positive and negative controls must also be run and tested.
- Incubation and washing is a must to get rid of unbound reagents at every step of this test.

Uses of ELISA Test

- It is very simple and sensitive test
- It requires very small quantity of test sample and other reagents

- It can be used to estimate qualitative and quantitative antigen, e.g. Hepatitis B surface antigen (HBsAg), rotavirus antigen, etc.
- It can be used to estimate qualitative and quantitative antibody, e.g. HIV antibody, mycobacterial antibody, etc.
- It is useful for diagnostic as well as epidemiological studies
- By doing, ELISA hormonal assay can also be done
- Unlike immunofluorescence test, ELISA is safe and less expensive.

ELISA Test for Hepatitis B Surface Antigen

1. Allow all the reagents to attain room temperature
2. Dilute concentrated washing solution 1/10 with distilled or deionized water
3. Gently mix all liquid reagents before use
4. Transfer 100 µl of each control, positive as well as negative and 100 µl of each test sample to the appropriate wells. Blank well is left empty
5. Cover the plate with an adhesive seal and incubate at 37°C for 1 hour
6. Remove the adhesive cover and discard it. Aspirate the contents of wells and add 300 µl diluted washing solution. Repeat this washing procedure 4 times.
7. Now add 100 µl of diluted conjugate to each well except blank control
8. Cover the plate with adhesive seal and incubate for 30 minutes at 37°C
9. Now prepare and dilute chromogen solution with substrate buffer
10. Remove and discard adhesive cover wash plate as mentioned in Step 6
11. Add 100 µl substrate—tetramethylbenzidine (TMB) to each well. Now incubate the plate uncovered at room temperature (25°C)
12. Now stop the reaction by adding 100 µl of 1 N sulfuric acid
13. Blank the reader at 450 nm with blank well and read the absorbance of each well in 30 minutes.

Results

Absorbance value of each sample is correlated with cut-off value. All the samples with an absorbance equal to or more than cut-off value should be declared positive for hepatitis B surface antigen.

SECTION 4

Hematology

Section Outline
- ❖ Hematology

CHAPTER 5

Hematology

Introduction

Hematology is the study of the blood which includes its cells and fluid surrounding them. The blood consists of pale yellow fluid called plasma which is a mixture of:
- Red blood cells also called erythrocytes.
- White blood cells also called leukocytes.
- Platelets also called thrombocytes.

The blood remains in motion continuously flowing through arteries carrying oxygenated blood from heart to various parts of the body by the pumping action of heart. Blood also flows through veins carrying deoxygenated blood (dark red) from different parts of the body to heart and to lungs. The arteries divide into smaller blood vessels called capillaries which supply blood to the various tissues. The capillaries then rejoin to form veins.

Plasma

Plasma contains proteins (albumin, globulin, prothrombin and fibrinogen). Albumin is water soluble which helps to control flow of water between the tissue fluid which surrounds the tissue cells and the blood.

Globulins include immunoglobulins which form defense antibodies.

Prothrombin and fibrinogen are made in liver and are blood clotting factors.

Plasma also contains electrolytes like potassium, sodium, calcium, magnesium, carbonates, bicarbonates, chlorides, etc. Electrolytes help to keep the blood at correct pH, i.e. 7.35 to 7.40.

Functions of Blood
- It helps to carry oxygen to all parts of the body by means of hemoglobin of red blood cells.

- It takes hormones from the glands of the body to other parts of the body where they are required to act
- It takes digested food material and vitamins to the body cells.
- It carries antibodies to various parts of the body
- It helps to remove the waste products, e.g. carbon dioxide, urea, etc.
- It helps in the defense of the body against bacteria and other harmful material which may enter the body. This is mainly done by leukocyte cells (white blood cells).

Red Blood Cells (Erythrocytes)

Shape (Fig. 5.1A)

- Round cells filled with hemoglobin
- When seen from their side they look like biconcave
- Do not contain nuclei.

Size: 7.5 μ

Number: 50,00,000 per cu mm of blood.

White Blood Cells (Leukocytes)

Shape (Fig. 5.1B)

Round, each containing nucleus and few granules.

Size: 9 to 20 μ.

Number: 4 to 7000 per cu mm of blood.

Platelets (Thrombocytes)

Shape (Fig. 5.1C)

Fragments of cells of various shapes, i.e. triangular, star, oval, etc. with granules.

Size: 2 to 5 μ.

Number: 3,00,000 per cu mm of blood

Function: Clotting of blood.

Chapter 5: Hematology

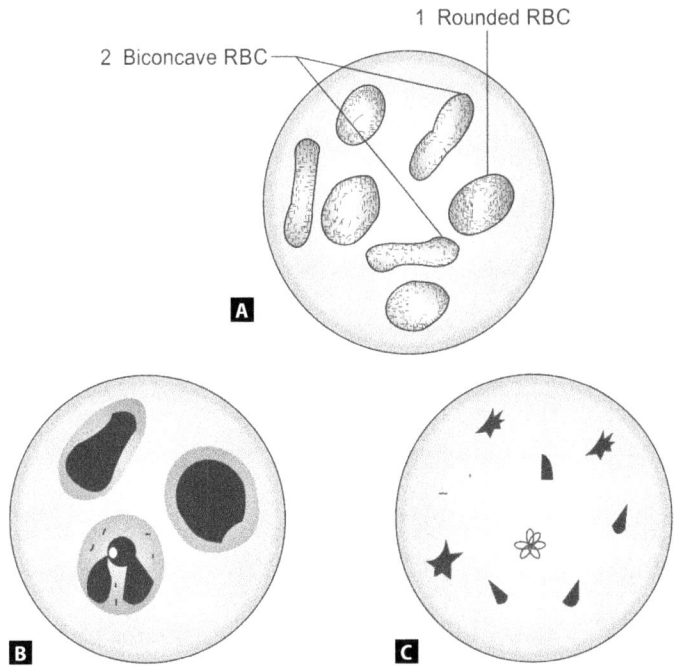

Figs 5.1A to C: (A) Red blood cells; (B) White blood cells; (C) Platelets thrombocytes

Estimation of Hemoglobin

Sahli's Acid Hematin Method

Principle: Hemoglobin is changed into acid hematin by hydrochloric acid. The brown color of the compound formed is matched with a brown glass standard in a comparator.

Requirements (Fig. 5.2)

Sahli's hemoglobinometer consists of (**Figs 5.3A to I**):
- Comparator with glass standard.
- A square hemoglobin tube marked both in grams and percentage figures.
- Hemoglobin pipette marked at 20 cu mm.
- 0.1 N HCl.

Section 4: Hematology

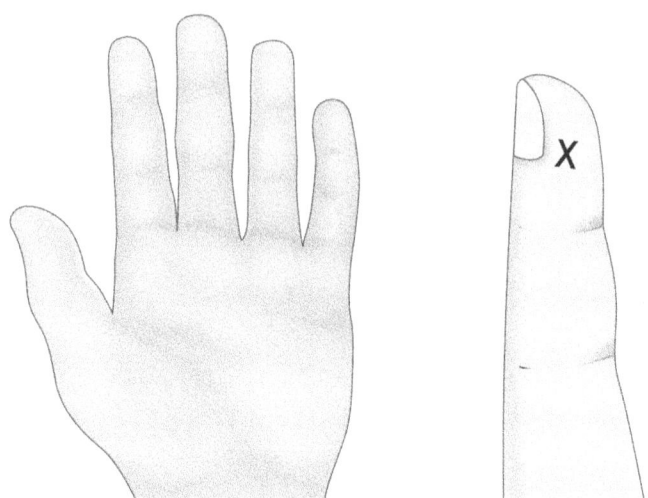

Fig. 5.2: Best site of finger prick is 3rd and 4th finger of left hand. At the side of finger which is less sensitive than tip

Procedure

- Fill the hemoglobin calibrated tube up to mark 20 with 0.1 N HCl by means of a dropper.
- Fill the hemoglobin pipette exactly upto 20 cu mm mark by gentle controlled sucking. The pipette is held horizontally while taking the blood. Wipe off with gauge, the blood on the outside of pipette.
- Empty this pipette into the acid in the tube by keeping the point of pipette to the bottom of the tube and gently blowing off the blood without causing bubbles.
- Rinse this pipette at least 3 times by drawing in and discharging the blood acid mixture.
- Mix the acid hematin solution in the tube with glass rod and allow the tube to stand for 10 minutes.
- Now dilute the solution of acid hematin by adding distilled water, drop by drop, keep on stirring the mixture all the time with glass rod.
- The comparator is held against good daylight and continue adding water, till color of solution matches perfectly with that of the standard.
- Record the reading in grams percent.

Chapter 5: Hematology

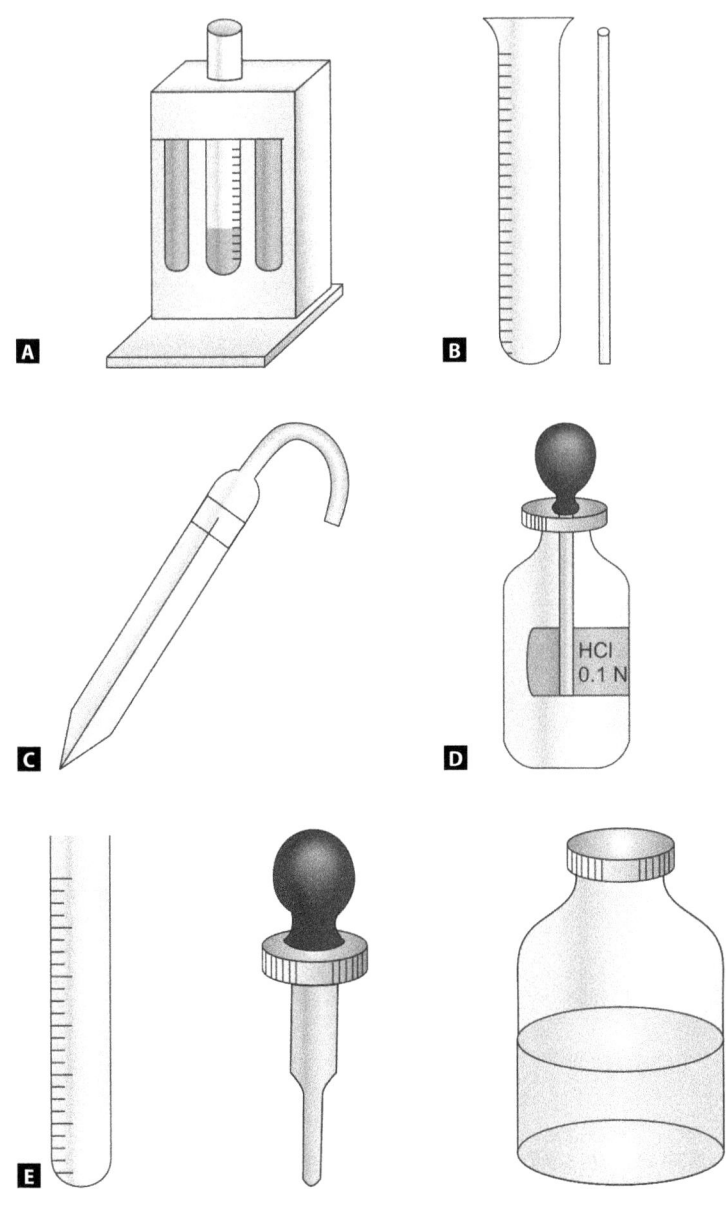

(Figs 5.3A to E)

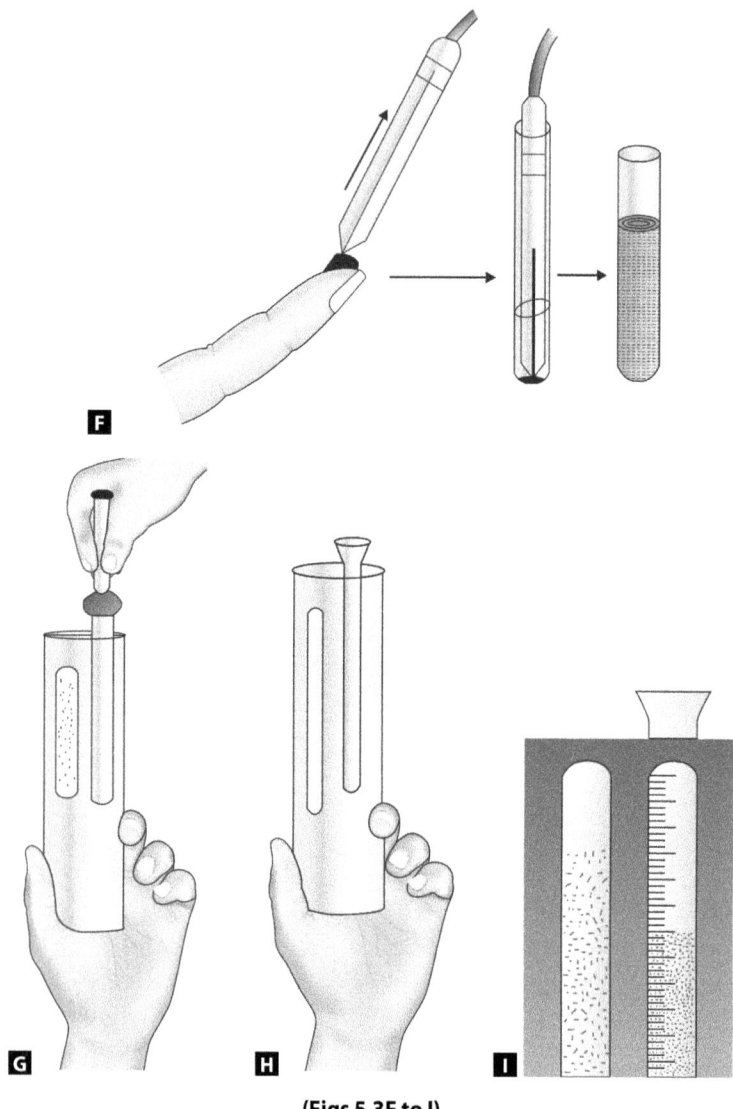

(Figs 5.3F to I)

Figs 5.3A to I: (A) Sahli's hemoglobinometer; (B) Glass rod and tube; (C) Sahli's pipette; (D) HCl bottle; (E) Pour 0.1N HCl upto 20 mark in tube; (F) Blood to be filled in pipette (Sahli's) upto 0.02 ml; (G) Place graduated tube in hemoglobinometer; (H) Add distilled water, if required; (I) Compare the color of the tube containing diluted blood with color of reference tube

Cyanmethemoglobin Method

Principle

Potassium ferricyanide changes hemoglobin from ferrous to ferric form. The methemoglobin formed reacts with potassium cyanide to produce stable pigment called cyanmethemoglobin.

Requirements

- Photoelectric calorimeter with filter 540 nm
- Test tubes
- Pipettes of 5 ml capacity
- Micropipettes 20 µl (if not available Sahli's pipette may be used)
- Drabkin's solution.

Calibration curve: Hemoglobin standard for cyanmethemoglobin method is used for calibrating. Take 3 dry and clean test tubes and proceed as under:
1. Pipette 5 ml of hemoglobin standard in the first tube (60 mg/100 ml).
2. In the second tube, measure exactly 2.5 ml of hemoglobin standard plus 2.5 ml of hemoglobin diluting reagent. Stopper the tube and mix well. This is 1:1 dilution of standard (30 mg cyanmethemoglobin per 100 ml).
3. In the third tube, add 5 ml of hemoglobin diluting reagent which acts as blank.

Measurement of optical density-cum-transmittance:
- First of all, set the wavelength of photoelectric colorimeter at 540 nm. Pour the blank (test tube no. 3) into the cuvette. See the optical density to zero or transmission at 100 percent.
- Pour the diluted hemoglobin standard (test tube no. 2) into the cuvette and record the optical density or percent transmission (cyanmethemoglobin standard).
- Pour undiluted hemoglobin standard into cuvette and record the optical density or percent transmission.
- Plot a graph for hemoglobin in mg/dl on horizontal axis and optical density on vertical axis.
- The equivalent gm/dl hemoglobin estimation/concentration in undiluted and diluted standard can be calculated as under:
  - gm/dl hemoglobin value of undiluted standard × dilution factor
  - 0.06 × 251 (if the concentration of hemoglobin standard is 60 mg/dl)

- 15.06 gm/dl hemoglobin value of 1:1 diluted standard
- gm/dl hemoglobin value of diluted standard × dilution factor
- 0.03 × 251 (half concentration of the hemoglobin standard 60 mg/ml)
- 7.53 = 7.5
- The mg/dl hemoglobin value (printed on the label) divided by 1000 gives the gm/dl hemoglobin.
- The procedure using 0.02 ml of whole blood in 5 ml of hemoglobin diluting reagent, the dilution factor is 251.
- Draw a straight line connecting the 2 plotted point on the graph which should pass through origin.

Procedure

	Test	Blank
Hemoglobin reagent	5 ml	5 ml
Fresh blood (whole)	0.02 ml	—

- Mix well, allow the stand at room temperature for 3 minutes.
- Measure optical density-cum transmittance of test against blank at 540 nm.

Recording of Readings

- From optical density reading of test specimen find concentration of hemoglobin in gm/dl with the help of calibration curve.
- In case the single standard reading is taken the following calculation method is used:

Hemoglobin = Optical density of unknown sample of blood/optical density of standard × concentration of standard in mg/dl × dilution factor gm/dl/1000.

Example

$$\frac{0.385 \times 60 \times 251 \times 1000}{0.418} = 13.8 \text{ gm/dl}$$

- Alternatively, we can calculate as under:
  - If optical density reading of test specimen is 0.385.
  - From optical density index of 0.385, draw a straight line parallel to the horizontal axis until it crosses the calibration curve.

- From this crossed point, draw a line parallel to vertical axis down to horizontal axis and calculate the value accordingly.

NORMAL RANGE OF HEMOGLOBIN

Men	15.5 gm/dl
Women	14 gm/dl
Infants (full-term cord blood)	16.5 gm/dl
Children 3 months	11 gm/dl
Children 3 to 6 years	12 gm/dl
Children 10 to 12 years	13 gm/dl

Total Red Blood Cell Count

Specimen (Fig. 5.4)

It can be done on an oxalated blood or capillary blood directly collected into pipette.

Requirements (Figs 5.5A to D)

- Red blood cell pipette.
- Diluting fluid (40% formaldehyde) 10 ml trisodium citrate (3% w/v).
- Neubauer's chamber
- Coverslip.

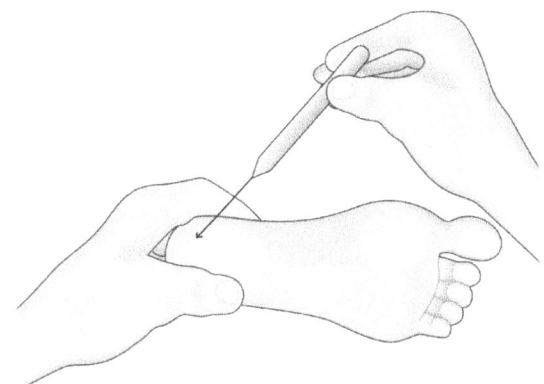

Fig. 5.4: Prick the heel of big toe in babies under 6 months

Section 4: Hematology

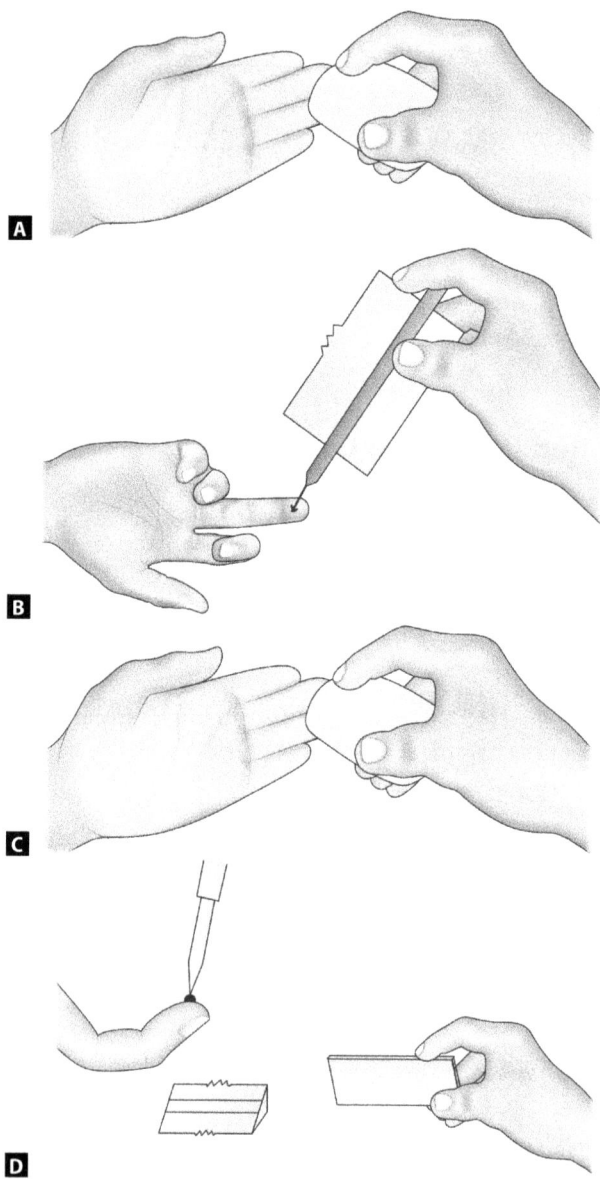

Figs 5.5A to D: (A) Clean the site of prick with cotton soaked in spirit; (B) Prick the finger end rapidly; (C) Wipe away the first drop of blood with dry cotton swab; (D) After pricking, collect the blood in a pipette or clean glass slide

Procedure

- Fill the red blood cell pipette upto 0.5 mark by holding the pipette horizontally. Use only clean and dry pipette.
- Draw diluting fluid up to the mark 101 (dilution 1:200).
- While filling the bulb, pipette should be gently rotated to obtain good mixture.
- Coverslip is placed over clean, grease-free and dry Neubauer's chamber. Coverslip should cover both ruled platforms.
- Now load the Neubauer's chamber as under:
  - Mix well the contents of red blood cell pipette for about 3 minutes.
  - Discard about 6 drops from pipette which may contain unmixed fluid with blood.
  - Hold the pipette at 45°C and release a drop of blood mixture by touching the space between the coverslip and chamber by the point of pipette.
  - Allow the mixture to run under the coverslip. It should be just sufficient to cover whole ruled platform. There should not be air- bubbles.
- Wait for 2 minutes for setting the cells.
- Counting of red blood cells is done as under:
  - In RBC count, the central double ruled square is used. Red blood cells are 80 very small squares have to be counted.
  - These 80 small squares comprise of 5 medium-sized squares, each of which is bound by triple line. Usually, they are four corners squares and one central square.

Calculation

Total area of the whole large central square = 1 sq mm
The smallest square has side of 1/20 mm so the area = 1/400 sq mm.
As depth in 1/10 mm, its volume = 1/4000 cu mm
Total volume of 80 small squares is 80/4000 = 1/50 cu mm
Dilution is 1:200
RBC count = Dilution × 1/Volume × Number of cells counted (N)
   = 200 × 50 × N = 10,000 × N cells/cu mm

Normal Values

4.5 – 5.9 million/cu mm

Erythrocyte Sedimentation Rate

Principle

When anticoagulant is added to the blood sample and then allowed to stand in a tube, the red cells slowly settle down to the bottom of tube leaving clear plasma above. The rate of sedimentation, estimated under standard conditions, is called erythrocyte sedimentation rate (ESR).

Procedure (Figs 5.6A to K)

ESR can be done by two methods.

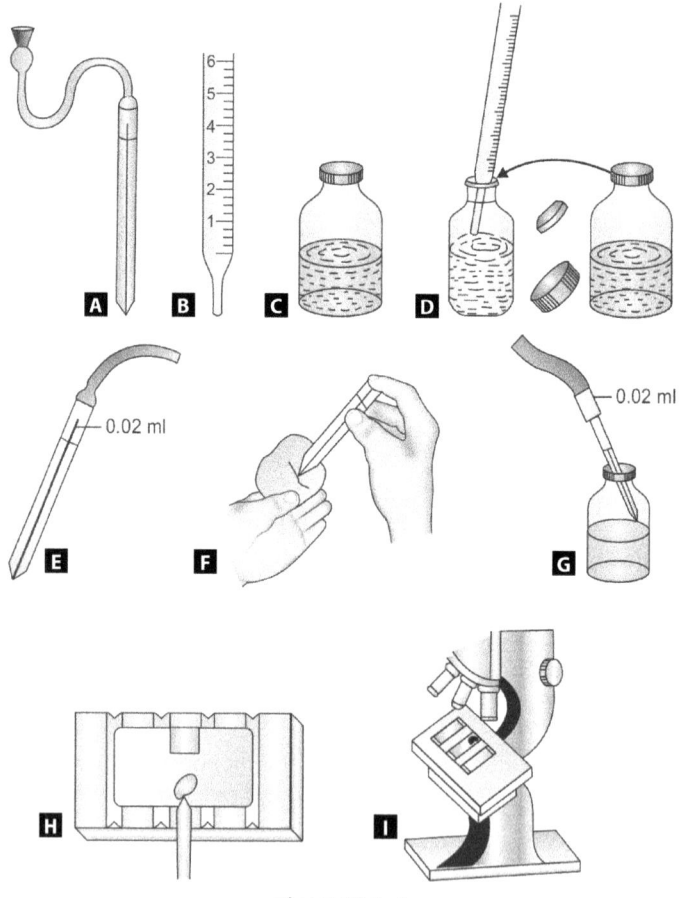

Figs 5.6A to I

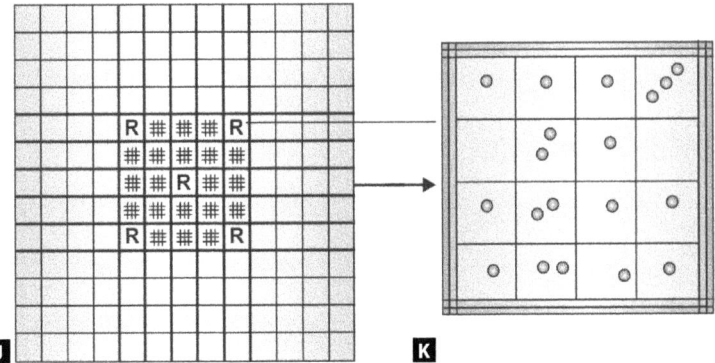

Figs 5.6J and K

Figs 5.6A to K: Red blood cell count (A) Blood pipette; (B) Graduated 5 ml pipette; (C) Empty bottle; (D) Add 4 ml diluting fluid; (E) Draw 0.02 ml of blood; (F) Wipe the outside of pipette with absorbent paper; (G) Blow the blood into bottle; (H) With pasture pipette fill two ruled areas of chamber (I) Count under microscope RBC settle on. Charged Neubauer's chamber; (J) Count red blood cells on; (K) Neubauer's counting chamber

Wintrobe Method

Requirements (Figs 5.7A to C)
- Wintrobe tube with following features:
  - Length 110 mm
  - Diameter 3 mm
  - Graduation of lower 100 mm from 0 to 100.
- *Anticoagulant*: Sodium citrate (0.4 ml)

Procedure
- Tube is filled up to 100 mm mark
- It is allowed to stand in vertical condition at room temperature
- Read the fall of red cells at the end of 1 hour.

Uses
- It can be used to find packed cell volume
- Buffy coat can be prepared.

Normal Values

Men   : 0 to 9 mm in first hour
Women : 0 to 20 mm in first hour.

Section 4: Hematology

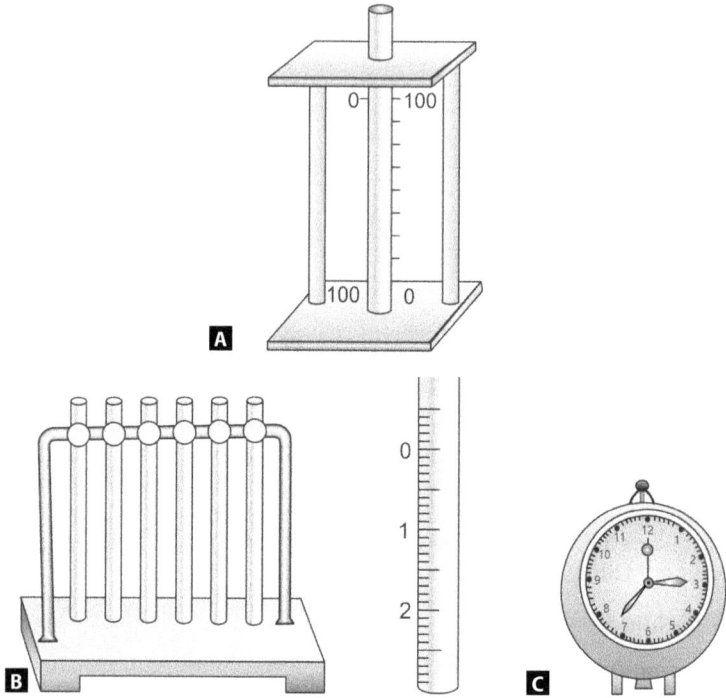

Figs 5.7A to C: (A) Wintrobe's ESR tube; (B) Six tubes with stand; (C) Graduation on Wintrobe's tube

Westergren Method (Figs 5.8A and B)

Requirements

- Westergren tube with following features:
  - Length 300 mm
  - Diameter 2.5 mm
  - Graduation in mm from 0 to 200.
- *Anticoagulant*: 0.5 ml (3.13% sodium citrate solution).

Procedure

- The blood mixture (blood + coagulant) drawn into Westergren tube up to the zero mark.
- Tube is set upright in a stand with a spring clip on top and rubber at bottom.
- The level of the top red cell is read at the end of one hour.

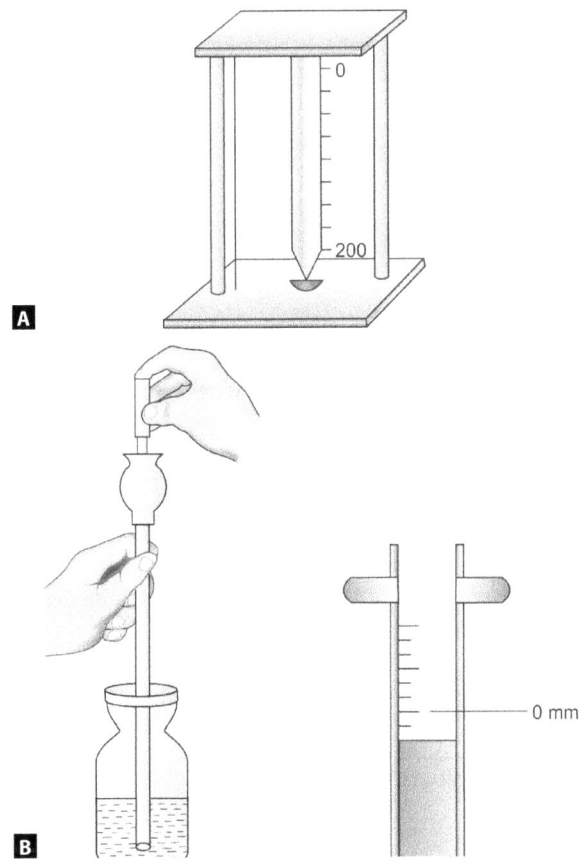

Figs 5.8A and B: (A) Westergren ESR pipettes stand; (B) Draw-citrated blood into Westergren pipette (using rubber bulb) upto 0 mark

Normal Values (Fig. 5.9)

Men   : 0 to 10 mm in first hour
Women : 0 to 20 mm in first hour.

Packed Cell Volume (PCV)
Procedure
- With the help of capillary pipette, a Wintrobe's hematocrit tube is filled upto 100 mark with anticoagulated blood, 0.5 ml blood contains 4 mg potassium oxalate and 6 mg ammonium oxalate.

Section 4: Hematology

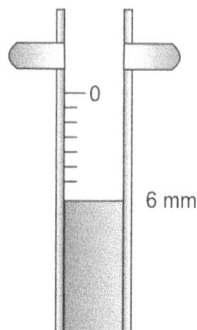

Fig. 5.9: After 1 hour note the height of the column of plasma in mm graduation (0 mark at the top of tube)

- It is centrifuged at 2500 revolutions per minute for 30 minutes.
- Note down the level of packed cells.
- Keep on centrifuging for 5 minutes time and note the level of packed cell, till packed cells show same level.
- PCV can be used directly or as a percentage as height of column of red cells in the tube is 100 mm.
- Above red cells is a grayish-red layer of leukocytes and above it is a buffy coat.

$$PCV\% = \frac{\text{Packed RBC column height}}{\text{Total blood column height}} \times 100$$

Normal Values

Men : 47%
Women : 42%

Absolute Values and Color Index

Mean Corpuscular Volume (MCV)

$$MCV = \frac{PCV\ \% \times 1000}{\text{Red blood cells (RBC) per cubic mm}}$$

$$\text{or } MCV = \frac{PCV\ (L/L) \times 1000}{RBC\ (10^{12}/L)}$$

Normal value: 78 to 94 cu mm

Raised value: Macrocytic anemia (MCV above 100 cubic microns)

Reduced value: Microcytic hypochromic anemia (below 80 cu microns)

Mean Corpuscular Hemoglobin (MCH)

$$MCH = \frac{Hb \text{ (g per 100 ml)} \times 100}{RBC \text{ count million/cu mm}}$$

Normal value: 27 to 32 pg per cell

Raised value: Macrocytic anemia

Reduced value: Hypochromic anemia

Mean Corpuscular Hemoglobin Concentration (MCHC)

$$MCHC = \frac{Hemoglobin \text{ per 100 ml blood}}{Packed \text{ cell volume (PCV)\%}} \times 100$$

Normal value: 32 to 38%

Raised value: Iron deficiency anemia and macrocytic anemia

Increased value: It cannot be more than 38% as the red cell stroma cannot hold a greater than normal concentration of hemoglobin.

Color Index

$$Color \text{ index} = \frac{Hemoglobin \text{ as percentage (14.5 gm hemoglobin as 100\%)}}{Red \text{ blood cells expressed as a percentage of normal (50,00,000 as 100\%)}}$$

Example

If hemoglobin is 60% and RBC count is 4,00,000, then color index is 60/4/5 × 100 = 60 × 5/4 × 100 = 0.75

Normal value: 0.9 to 1.1

Raised values: Pernicious anemia

Reduced values: Iron deficiency anemia

Section 4: Hematology

Total Leukocyte Count

Specimen: Leukocyte count may be done on EDTA blood or capillary blood.

Requirements (Figs 5.10A to I)

- A white blood cell pipette **(Fig. 5.10A)**.
- Diluting fluid containing:
  - 2% acetic acid
  - 2 drops of gentian violet per liter

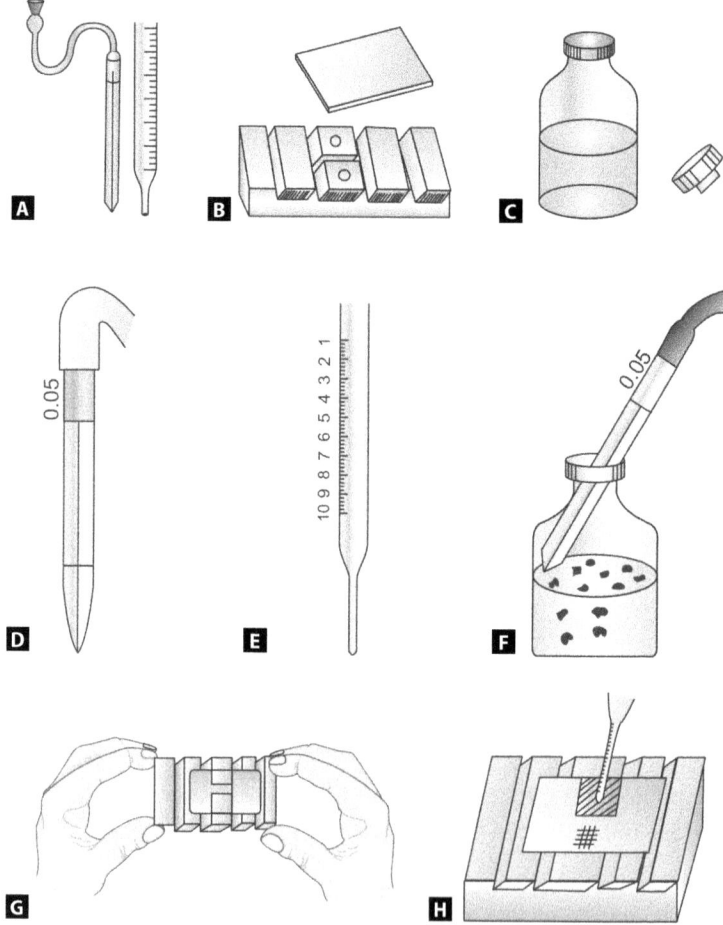

Figs 5.10A to H

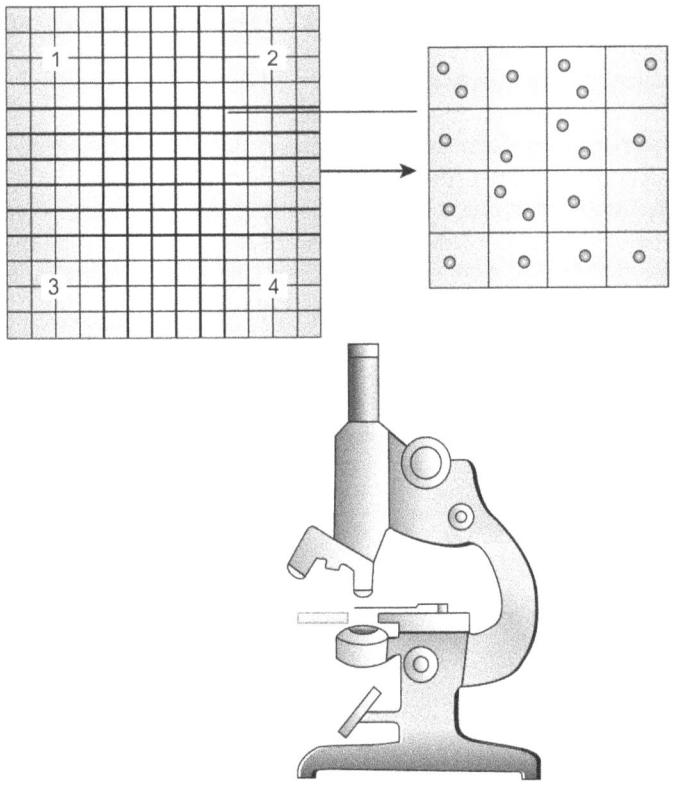

Fig. 5.10I

Figs 5.10A to I: Total leukocyte count: (A) WBC pipette graduated to 0.05 ml and graduated pipette 1 ml and graduated pipette 1 ml; (B) Neubauer ruled counting chamber and special coverslip; (C) Pipette 0.95 ml of diluting fluid in small bottle; (D) Draw 0.05 ml blood; (E) Wipe outside of pipette with absorbent paper; (F) Blow the 0.05 ml blood into bottle containing diluting fluid; (G) Attach the cover glass to Neubauer's chamber; (H) Fill the Neubauer's chamber with diluted blood using Pasteur pipette; (I) Counting of leukocytes as shown (1, 2, 3, 4)

- Neubauer's chamber with cover glass **(Fig. 5.10B)**.
- Microscope.

Procedure

- Take blood in a clean dry pipette up to the mark 0.5.
- Wipe off the outside of the pipette with gauze.

- Now take the diluting fluid upto 11 (dilution 1 to 20). Keep on rotating the pipette slowly.
- Mix well the contents of pipette.
- Discard first few drops from pipette.
- Take clean, dry Neubauer's chamber and place cover glass. Both ruled platforms should be properly covered with cover glass.
- By holding the pipette at 45°C and touching the space between cover glass and the Neubauer's chamber by the point of pipette, put a drop of mixture which spreads under the cover glass by capillary actions. There should not be any air bubble.
- Wait for 2 minutes for setting of cells.
- The counting of leukocytes is done under low power of microscope.
- Bring one of the four corner squares into the field.
- Reduce light and count number of brown dots seen.
- Count such cells in all four squares (**Figs 5.10C to I**).
- Total them up.

Calculation

The area of each large squares = 1 sq mm

Normal Range

Adults: 4,500-11,000/cu mm
Neonates: 10,000-25,000/ cu mm
Volume of square = 0.1 cu mm
Volume of 4 corner squares = 0.1 × 4 = 0.4 cu mm
Number of cells in 4 corner squares = N
0.4 cu mm contains N cells
1 cu mm contains N × 20/0.4 (dilution factor) = N × 50

Differential Leukocyte Count

- This is done in well-prepared film, the cells running in strips whole length of the film (**Fig. 5.11**).
- It should be examined using oil immersion objective.
- At least, 200 cells should be counted.

Preparation of Film

- Take a drop of blood and place it in central line of a slide about 1 to 2 cm from one end of the slide (**Fig. 5.12A**).

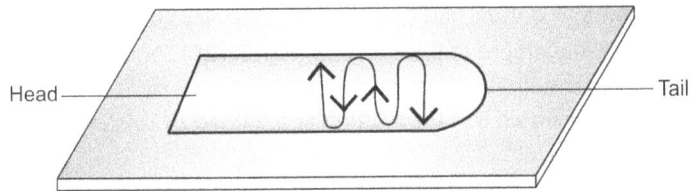

Fig. 5.11: Ideal blood smear

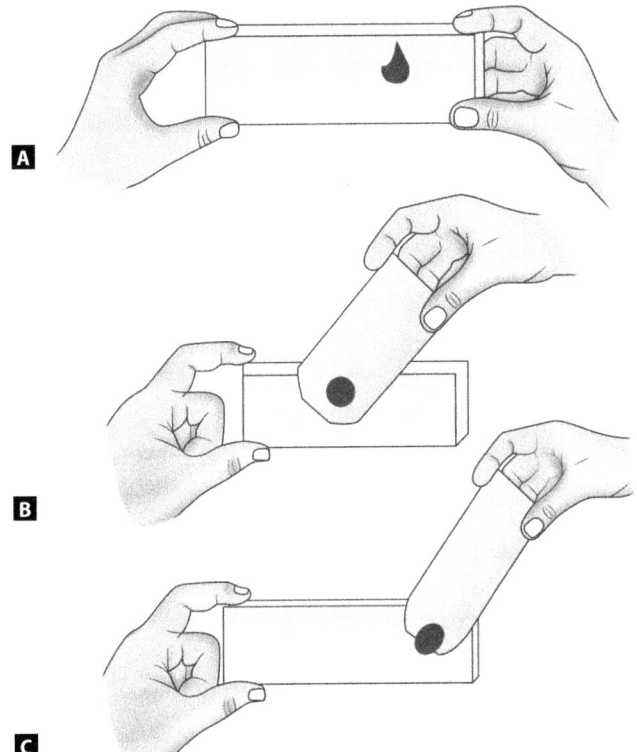

Figs 5.12A to C: Differential leukocytic count (DLC) (A) Collection of drop of blood and touch it lightly with one end of slide; (B) Placing of edge of spreader just in front of drop of blood; (C) Spreader is moved back until it touches drop of blood

- The spreader is placed at an angle of 45°C to the slide and then moved back to make contact with the drop (**Fig. 5.12B**).
- The drop should spread quickly along the line of contact of spreader with the slide.

- As soon as it occurs, film should be spread very rapidly by smooth, forward movement of the spreader (**Fig. 5.12C**)
- The drop should be of such size that the film is 3 to 4 cm in length.
- The smear should be rapidly dried and stained by Leishman's stain.

Procedure of Leukocyte Count

- Cells should be counted using oil immersion objective.
- Cell should be counted in a strip of film running the whole length.
- The lateral edges of film are avoided.
- The film should be inspected from head to tail.
- At least, 200 cells should be counted.

Leishman's Stain (Figs 5.13A to G)

Dissolve 0.15% Leishman's stain in methyl alcohol.

Procedure of Leishman's Staining

- Put sufficient stain solution on smear to cover it fully.
- Wait for 2 minutes.
- Add twice the quantity of buffer to stain.
- Avoid overflow and suck the mixture in and out with the pipette to ensure thorough mixing. A scum will form on the smear.
- All this diluted stain is to act for 5 minutes.
- Wash the smear.
- Wipe to clean the back of the smear and allow it to dry and see it under microscope (oil immersion).

Types of Leukocytes seen in Normal Blood (Fig. 5.14)

Neutrophils Polymorphonuclear Cells

- Multilobed nucleus
- Normal range is 50 to 70%.

Eosinophil Cells

- Bilobed nucleus.
- Coarse oxyphil bright red granules.
- The normal range is 0 to 3%.

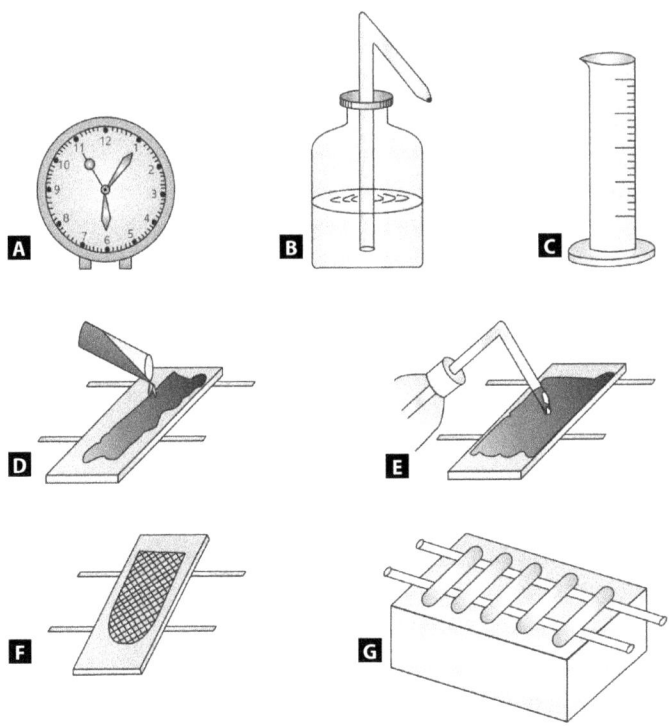

Figs 5.13A to G: Leishman's staining of blood smear (A) Timer clock; (B) Wash bottle; (C) Measuring cylinder; (D) Two glass rods over staining tank; (E) Cover the slide with Leishman's stain for 2 to 3 minutes; and (F and G) Allow the stained slide to dry in a slide rack and slide box

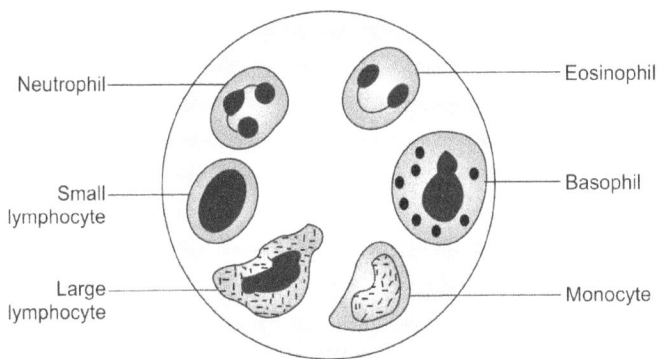

Fig. 5.14: Peripheral blood film (PBF): Neutrophil, small lymphocyte, large lymphocyte, eosinophil, basophil, monocyte

Basophil Cells

- Bilobed nucleus
- Coarse basophilic granules
- Normal value 0 to 1%.

Monocyte Cells

- Kidney-shaped nucleus
- Bluish gray cytoplasm
- Normal value is 2 to 8%.

DLC Values

- Neutrophils—40–75%
- Lymphocytes—20–40%
- Eosinophils—1–6%
- Monocytes—2–10%
- Basophils—0–1%

Lymphocyte Cells

- Rounded nucleus
- Rim of strongly basophilic cytoplasm
- Normal values 15 to 40%

Reticulocyte Count

Reticulocytes are young red cells which contain basophilic ribonucleoprotein but no nucleus.

Requirements

- *Staining solution*:
    - Brilliant cresyl blue — 1 gm
    - 3% sodium citrate — 20 ml
    - 0.9% NaCl — 80 ml
    - First dissolve dye in and then add sodium. Mix and filter the stain and store at room temperature.
- Small test tube
- Anticoagulant (oxalated or EDTA)
- Thermometer
- Slide

- Microscope
- Incubator.

Procedure

- Take 3 to 4 drops of staining solution in a small tube
- Add equal amount of oxalated or EDTA blood
- Mix well and keep it in an incubator at 37°C for 15 to 20 minutes
- Now gently mix the solution and prepare smears on slide.
- Smears are examined under microscope under oil immersion.

Calculation

- Count 100 reticulocytes
- For example, if

Number of reticulocytes in 150 fields = 100
Total number of red cells in 150 fields = 3000

$$\text{Reticulocyte (\%)} = \frac{100}{3000} \times 100 = 3.3\%$$

$$= \frac{\text{Number of reticulocytes}}{\text{Number of red cells + reticulocytes}} \times 100 = 3.3\%$$

Normal Value

Adult and children: 0.2 to 2%
Newborn infants: 2 to 6%

Absolute Eosinophil Count

Requirements

Eosinophil diluting fluid (Dunger's solution)

Stock Solution

Eosin yellow = 0.5 gm
Formaldehyde (40%) = 0.5 ml
Phenol (95%) aqueous = 0.5 ml
Distilled water up to = 100 ml

Working solution: Dilute 6 ml of stock solution with distilled water upto 100 ml.
- WBC pipette
- Neubauer's counting chamber

Procedure

- Suck blood up to 0.5 mark in a WBC pipette
- Dilute it up to 11 mark with diluting fluid
- Gently rotate the pipette
- Discard 3 to 4 drops of fluid
- Charge the Neubauer's counting chamber and allow it to stand for 3 minutes for the cells to settle down
- Count all the eosinophils in the whole of the ruled area (i.e. 9 squares).

Calculation

Absolute eosinophil count = $N \times 1/\text{Volume} \times \text{dilution}$
Volume = Length × Breadth × Depth
$\quad\quad = 3 \times 3 \times 0.1 = 0.9$ mm
$\quad\quad = N \times 1/0.9 \times 20$
$\quad\quad = N \times 10/9 \times 20 = N \times 200/9$
$\quad\quad = N \times 22.2/\text{cu mm}$

Normal value: 40 to 400 cells/cu mm.

Platelet Count

Specimen: Blood may be collected by clean puncture of vein and shifting it carefully into a tube containing anticoagulant dipotassium EDTA.

Requirements

- Dry RBC pipette
- Diluting fluid (Rees Ecker)

Ammonium oxalate 10 gm/l (1%), prepare freshly just before use
    Sodium citrate   3.8 gm
    Brilliant cresyl blue   0.05 gm
    Neutral formalin   0.65 ml
    Distilled water   0.100 ml
    Filter and centrifuge it at 2800 revolution per minute and store

- Centrifuge machine
- Neubauer's chamber
- Filter paper

Procedure

- Take blood in RBC pipette upto mark 0.5
- Wipe off the outside of the pipette
- Draw the working diluting fluid upto 101
- Shake the pipette for 5 minutes
- Discard the first 4 drops
- *Load the chamber*: Both the hemocytometer and the coverslip. Both of them must be dry and clean before use.
- All this preparation to stand for 15 minutes in a moist chamber.
- Count platelets under high power. Platelets are lilac colored. Count at least 300 platelets and calculate as under. Calculate in the four large corner squares (4 mm^2).

Calculation

$$\frac{\text{Number of platelets counted} \times 10 \times \text{dilution}}{\text{Number of 1 square counted}} = \text{Platelets/cu mm}$$

$$\frac{10 \times 200}{4} = 500 \text{ Platelets/cu mm}$$

Normal value: 1,50,000 to 4,00,000 cells/cu mm

Coagulation Time

Principle: A measure of time required for blood to solidify (coagulate) after it has been removed from the body.

Capillary Method

Requirements

- Pricking needle
- Spirit lamp
- Stop watch
- Capillary tube.

Procedure

- Prick the fingertip and draw blood up in a capillary tube 1 mm in diameter
- Start the stop watch
- After every 30 seconds break a short segment of tube until a coagulated thread appears.

Normal value: 3 to 5 minutes

Lee and White Method

Requirements

- Standard size tubes
- Thermometer
- Pricking needle
- Spirit lamp.

Procedure

- Blood is poured in 4 standard size tubes
- Keep these tubes at 37°C
- Start the stop watch right at the moment prick is given
- Time when the tube can be tilted at 90° without spilling the blood is noted
- Coagulation time is the time from the moment of puncture to the average time at which the tubes can be tilted to an angle more than 90° without spilling the blood.

Normal value: 6 to 9 minutes.

Interpretation: Coagulation time is more than normal in:
- Hemophilia
- If person has taken anticoagulant drugs.

Coagulation time is less than normal in:
- Typhoid fever
- After bleeding
- In heart diseases namely endocarditis
- After removal of spleen
- After taking food
- After giving anesthesia (before operation).

Bleeding Time (Duke's Method)

Procedure

- Stab the fingertip with sterilized needle
- Blot off the drop of blood every 30 seconds until it stops to ooze from stab prick of fingertip.
- Blots are recorded in series along a strip of blotting paper and later on counted.

Collection of Blood

Mainly, there are following two methods to collect blood samples:

Venous Blood

- It is preferred because a good number of tests can be done.
- To withdraw blood patient should ideally be in lying down position where adequate light is there.
- Make the veins of upper part of forearm (at elbow) prominent by applying tourniquet or blood pressure apparatus cuff kept at around 70 mm Hg.
- Ask the patient to open and close his hands several times to further making the vein prominent.
- Select the best vein which is both visible, can be felt and well fixed with surrounding tissue.
- The part from where blood is to be taken is cleaned with cotton moistened with spirit.
- Patient's forearm is grasped with washed and dry left hand to steady the vein.
- The thumb retracts downwards soft tissue below the site of puncture.
- The needle is brought to the skin over the vein, the bevel of the needle turned up.
- The skin is punctured first and vein next. The plunger is pulled back gently.
- When blood start flowing into syringe the tourniquet is released.
- After required blood is taken, the needle is withdrawn and punctured site is pressed with a swab of cotton moisture with spirit for 2 minutes.
- The patient is asked to elevate the arm and maintain pressure for few minutes more to prevent hematoma.

- Before putting blood in bottle or tube, the needle of syringe should be removed.
- Use the blood so collected for required test.

Capillary Blood

- It is obtained by pricking the skin.
- Only small quantity of blood (few drops) can be collected with this method.
- Blood is collected directly in pipettes and should be processed immediately.
- With this method following tests can be done:
  - Hemoglobin estimation
  - Red cell count
  - Leukocyte count
  - Platelet count
  - Reticulocyte count
  - For preparing smears for differential leukocytes count.

Technique

- Capillary blood is obtained from tips of fingers or lobe of the ear in case of adults. In case of infants, the sites are heel, ball of thumb, the great toe.
- The site of puncture is selected and cleaned with spirit and allow the part to dry completely.
- The point of sterilized needle is touched with the skin and bold quick prick is made.
- The prick should be 2 to 4 mm deep so that there is free-flow of blood.
- Blood must flow at once from the prick site.
- The first drop is wiped off.
- Second drop is collected for filling pipette or preparing smear on slide.
- Squeezing of punctured site is not allowed as it may dilute the blood with the tissue fluid.

Arterial Blood

Sometimes, it may be difficult to collect blood from veins. In such situations, arterial blood may be collected from brachial and radial

arteries in cases of subacute bacterial endocarditis, arterial blood culture tests positive even when venous blood culture shows no bacteria. Venous blood is necessary for following test:
- Estimation of ESR, PVC, etc.
- Estimation of blood constituents like sugar, urea, etc.
- Blood culture
- Serological test like antistreptolysin O (ASO), Widal, etc.
- Blood grouping, cross-matching and blood donation.

Anticoagulants

The anticoagulants which are in use are:
- Ethylenediamine tetra-acetic acid (EDTA) carries following features:
  - The sodium and potassium salts of EDTA are powerful anticoagulants.
  - EDTA acts by its chelating effect on the calcium molecules in blood.
  - Preserve cellular elements better than oxalate.
  - It can be used in following test:
    - Blood counts
    - ESR
    - PCV estimation
  - It is not used in the tests related to coagulation diseases.
  - It is also not suitable to use EDTA in prothrombin time.
- Ammonium and potassium oxalate mixture carries following figures:
  - It consists of mixture of 2 parts of potassium oxalate and 3 parts of ammonium oxalate.
  - Acts by chelating calcium.
  - May be used for blood chemistry and hematology tests.
- Trisodium citrate has following features:
  - It is an anticoagulant of choice in coagulation studies.
  - Acts by chelating calcium.
- Heparin has following features:
  - Acts by inhibiting thrombin and other stages of clotting.
  - Used in the concentration of 15 IU per ml of blood.
  - It does not change the size of red blood cells.
  - It is the best anticoagulant to use for osmotic fragility tests.
  - It is not as useful as EDTA for general blood tests.
- Acid citrate dextrose (ACD) solution has following features:
  - Main use in blood bank for preserving blood for transfusion.
  - Useful for enzyme studies.

- Its use is also found in studying of hemolytic processes.
- One ml of ACD solution is sufficient to prevent coagulation of 4 ml of blood.

Lupus Erythematosus (LE) Cell Phenomenon

It consists of demonstration of a characteristic inclusions containing cell, the LE cell and clumps of leukocytes around inclusion material. There are two methods to detect this phenomenon.

Direct Method

- The coagulated patient's blood is incubated for 2 hours at 37°C.
- Bottle containing patient's blood is shaken and clot is crushed with clean rod.
- Defibrinated blood is then centrifuged and film made from buffy coat.
- It is stained with Leishman's stain.
- Look for LE cells under oil immersion of microscope.

Indirect Method

- Patient's blood is incubated with a suspension of normal leukocytes.
- After incubation, clot is crushed with a clean glass rod.
- Defibrinated blood is then centrifuged and film is made from buffy coat.
- It is stained with Leishman's stain.
- Look for LE cells under oil immersion objective.

Fragility of Red Blood Cells for Hemolytic Disorders

Principle

The fragility of red blood cells is shown by their inability to resist hemolysis in diminishing strength of salt solutions.

Method

- Two rows of test tubes containing 5 ml of diluted buffered sodium chloride solution is taken in each.
- Range of sodium chloride dilution should be from 0.8 to 0.2%.

- To row I of tubes add a drop of patient's blood to each tube.
- To row II of tubes add a drop of normal blood to each tube.
- Shake the tubes and let them stand for sometime when intact RBCs start settling down.
- Hemolysis if present will be seen in the form of pinkish discoloration of fluid.

Normal value: 0.4% cells do not hemolyze upto a dilution of 03%.

Interpretation

- *Diminished fragility*:
  - Sickle cell anemia
  - Thalassemia
  - Polycythemia
  - Anemias where target cells are present.
- *Increased fragility*:
  - Hereditary spherocytosis
  - Acquired hemolytic anemia

Prothrombin Time

Principle

The concentration of prothrombin in the plasma is estimated by measuring the length of time taken for plasma to clot in the presence of an excess of thrombokinase and calcium ions.

Procedure

- Blood is taken from patient and transferred into an anticoagulant solution (which prevents its clotting by removing calcium ions), e.g. citrate or oxalate.
- Centrifuge the plasma.
- Thromboplastins and calcium chloride are added.
- Time taken for the plasma to clot is noted with stop watch.

Normal Value

12 to 14 seconds

Interpretation

Increased prothrombin time:
- Vitamin K deficiency in newborn
- Malabsorption
- Liver diseases
- Anticoagulant therapy.

Normal value: 12 to 15 seconds

Increased value: Thrombocytopenic purpura

Clot Retraction

Principle

When whole blood is allowed to clot, the early clot is composed of all elements of the blood. After some time, the clot reduces in mass and fluid serum is expressed from the clot. It is due to an action of platelets on fibrin.

Requirements

- Blood container
- Clean, dry plain glass, centrifuge tube
- Timer
- Water bath.

Procedure

- 5 ml blood is taken from patient.
- It is transferred to the centrifuge tube.
- Incubate at 37°C in vertical position.
- Record degree of retraction after 1, 2 and 4 hours.
- Degree and rate of retraction is noted and also discoloration of serum.

Normal value: 48 to 64% in 1 hour.

Bone Marrow Examination

It is the only method of correctly diagnosing diseases of blood.

Sites of Bone Marrow Aspiration

The following sites are selected for bone marrow aspiration:
- Sternum
- Iliac crest and upper end of tibia in children.

Requirements

- A special bone marrow needle (Salah or Klima needle) along with stilette
- Local anesthesia (Lignocaine)
- 2 to 5 ml syringe
- Glass slides
- Absolute methanol
- Formal ethanol.

Procedure

- The site of puncture is usually sternum. Sterilize the selected site with soap water, iodine and finally with alcohol
- The site is anesthetized locally using lignocaine
- Skin and subcutaneous tissues are punctured using sterilized bone biopsy and needly
- When needle reaches periosteum, guarded needle is pushed further about 5 mm. Now the needle is fixed tightly in position
- Now the needle is further pushed with boring motion into the cavity of bone
- The stilette is removed and well fitted 2 to 5 ml syringe is used
- About 0.3 ml of bone marrow contents are sucked
- Punctured site is properly sealed.

Preparation of the Film

- Film must be prepared from aspirated bone marrow material immediately
- Film may be fixed in methanol followed by staining with Giemsa method
- Further film may be fixed in formal ethanol for other cytochemical staining if required.

Examination of Bone Marrow Smear

- *Estimate of cellularity*: One can say that smear is rich in cells or relatively a cellular. It is done on the ratio of fat spaces and hemopoietically active parenchyma (normal 1.2 to 1.1)

- *Detailed cellular structure and cell composition*:
    - It is done by estimating differential count
    - M:E ratio is also estimated (normally 1.5:1 to 3:1)
- *Hemosiderin in bone marrow*:
    - It is done by Peris's method to estimate hemosiderin
    - Iron stores are determined
    - Iron stores are decreased in iron deficiency anemia
    - Hemosiderine is increased in hemosiderosis and hemochromatosis.

Bone Marrow Biopsy

It is indicated as:
- Repeated failure to obtain material by aspiration
- Evaluation of cellularity in pancytopenia
- Dry tap but there is doubt of leukemia.

SECTION 5

Blood Transfusion

Section Outline
- Preservation of Blood

CHAPTER 6

Preservation of Blood

Introduction

Blood bank is a compact unit where blood is taken from healthy donor, processed, stored and then issued to needy patients on the instructions of attending doctors. A very important thing which should be remembered is that blood stock of the blood bank has to be replaced every time a unit of blood is issued for the patient. Hence, encouragement should be given to the idea of donating blood for a patient by attendants or other volunteers before getting is issued for the patient. Practice of purchasing blood from professional donors should be discouraged and *never accepted*.

Misgiving about donation of blood should be explained as under:
- Only human blood can be transfused to patients.
- Only healthy donors are selected for blood donation. All necessary tests are done for this purpose.
- Human body contains about 5 to 6 liters of blood and only 300 ml blood is taken. This amount is replaced in 48 to 72 hours automatically.
- No special diet or bed rest is required after blood donation.
- Whole process of checking of donor and donation of blood takes at the most 20 to 30 minutes.

Organization of Blood Bank

Location
- Should be situated within the premises of hospital.
- Attendants and unconcerned hospital personnels should not be permitted inside the blood bank. It is to ensure proper grouping and cross-matching procedures. Any mistake may cost blood transfusion reactions.

Designing
It should have:
- *Reception room*: It has the provision of registration counter, doctor's cabin, a small side laboratory (for hemoglobin estimation and other

tests, like blood grouping) and proper seating arrangement for proposed donors.
- *Donation room*: It has comfortable beds for donors, sterile equipment for bleeding donor, refrigerator resuscitation equipment, etc.
- *Donors rest and refreshing room.*
- *Laboratory*: It has the provision of blood grouping of recipient, grouping and proper labeling of donated blood, cross-matching of patient blood against stored, freshly donated blood.
- *Room for preservation of blood.*
- *Immunolaboratory for testing donated blood for*:
    - Australia antigen (Hepatitis-B surface antigen)
    - Malaria
    - Syphilis (VDRL test)
    - AIDS (ELISA for human immunodeficiency virus called HIV)
    - HCV

Blood Transfusion

It is the study of blood groups, types and preparation of blood transfusion. It is also called immunohematology (body defenses against "outside substances", i.e. antigen through the development of antibodies).

Blood Grouping

The red blood cell has its surface variety of antigen glycolipids or glycoproteins. An antigen is a large protein or polysaccharide substance which when introduced into the body of other man, sensitizes that man to produce antibodies which can react with this antigen specifically.

ABO Blood Grouping System

All people can be divided into four major groups by mixing the blood cells with two different antisera (known as (i) anti-A antisera (ii) anti-B antisera). Four major blood groups are:
1. A group
2. B group
3. AB group
4. O group

Method of ABO Blood Grouping

Slide Method

- Take a clean glass slide bearing number.
- Take two drops of blood after a finger prick or from citrated blood, on two corners of slide.

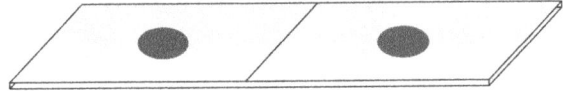

- On the left side, a drop of anti-A serum and on right side a drop of anti-B serum are added separately.

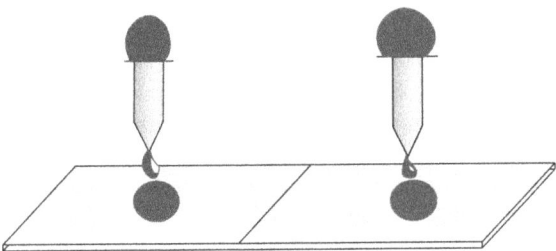

- The serum cell suspensions are mixed separately with the help of glass rod or by the corners of another glass slide.
- Tilt the slide with hand for 30 seconds to 1 minute.
- Result is noted on the appearance of clumps (curding) of red cells.
- Report the blood group as under:

Anti-sera		Conclusion	Result reportings
Anti-A sera	**Anti-B sera**		
Clumping	No clumping	'A' antigen on cell	'A' group
No clumping	Clumping	'B' antigen on cell	'B' group
Clumping	Clumping	Both 'A' and 'B' antigens on cell	'AB' group
No clumping	No clumping	Neither A nor B antigen on cell	'O' group

Tube Technique

- Mark two tubes with patient's number.
- Mark one tube anti A or just A and the other tube anti-B or B tube.

- Make 2% suspension in a saline of red blood cells.
- Add 2 drops of anti-A to tube A and 2 drops of anti-B to the tube marked B.
- Add 2 drops of cell suspension (2%) to each tube.
- Mix well and centrifuge both tubes at 1000 revolutions per minute for 1 minute.
- Remove the tubes and hold the tubes over concave mirror and inspect the deposited bottom of cells in the bottom.
- See agglutination and report as shown in above table.

Indirect Grouping

- Take 2 test tubes.
- Place 2 drops of patients sera into each of the 2 tubes.
- Add 2 drops of 2 to 5% suspension of group A cells in tube 1.
- Add 2 drops of 2 to 5% suspension of group B cells.
- Tubes are shaken and centrifuged at 1000 revolutions per minute for 1 minute.
- If clumping occurs in tube 1 and no clumping in tube 2, it belongs to blood group 'B'.
- If clumping occurs in tube 2 and no clumping in tube 1, then it is blood group 'A'.
- If there is clumping in tube 1 and tube 2, then it is blood group 'AB'.
- If no clumping occurs in tube 1 and tube 2, then it is blood group 'O'.

Rh Blood Grouping

The name Rh is taken from rhesus monkeys. First of all antibodies against RBCs of rhesus monkey were obtained by injecting monkey RBCs into rabbits and guinea-pigs.

Technique of Rh Grouping

Slide Test

- One drop of 40% cell suspension of patient on a clean slide is taken.
- Add 1 drop of anti-D sera to it.
- Mix them and look for clumping, if blood sample in Rh-positive.

Tube Test

- Take 1 drop of 5% cell suspension of patient in a tube.
- Add drop of anti-D sera to it.

- Centrifuge at 1000 revolutions per minute for one minute.
- Look for clumping with naked eye and microscope.

Selection of Blood Donors

- *Age*: Blood can be donated by person from 16 to 60 years.
- *Weight and height*: A person with a 5 feet height and 55 kg weight, can donate blood.
- *Frequency of blood donation*: Once in 3 months.
- *Hemoglobin levels*: About 12.5 g/dl.
- *Blood pressure*: A person with 110 to 140 mm Hg.
- *Pulse*: A person with 72 to 100 per minute.
- *Temperature*: It should be of 98°F to 98.6°F.
- *Vaccination*:
    - Those having received killed vaccine like cholera should donate blood, 1 week after vaccination.
    - Those having received live vaccine-like BCG should donate blood 3 weeks after vaccination.
    - Those who have received antisera like ATS, ADS, etc., should donate blood after 4 weeks.
- *Drugs*: All those receiving drugs for epilepsy, hypertension, etc., should not donate blood.
- Persons who are having asthma, allergy, tuberculosis, etc., should not donate blood.

Collection of Blood

- Let the donor lie comfortably on bed.
- Make the donor to feel at home and prepare him mentally and physically for blood donation.
- Ask the donor to relax and put a towel under the arm to be bled.
- In the mean time also tie a label to the ACD solution bottle that is going to have blood. Write down the name of the donor, blood group, date of collection and also date of expiry, i.e. 21 days.
- Tie a sphygmomanometer cuff around the donor's upper arm and pump it up to 60 mm Hg.
- Choose a large straight prominent vein.
- Clean the place over the choosen vein with a swab-soaked in spirit from middle outwards.
- Repeat the cleaning with swab soaked in iodine as described above.

- Finally, cleaning is done with swab soaked with spirit.
- Lignocaine may be injected locally near the proposed site of vein to be punctured.
- Now clamp the blood donor set with a forcep near the bottle and push the needle meant for blood collecting bottle, into the bottle.
- Now hold the needle meant for vein puncture, between your finger and thumb by the adopter with bevel upward.
- Push the needle through skin into the vein of arm of donor.
- As soon as blood is seen coming in the upper end of the tube, release the clamp by removing the forcep.
- Fix the needle to patient's arm by means of adhesive plaster.
- Gently mix the bottle and the ACD solution as blood collection bottle starts filling by constant gently shaking the bottle.
- If blood stops coming into the bottle, put in an airway into the bottle stopper of blood collecting bottle. Flow of blood into the bottle will start.
- After collecting about 300 ml blood (300 ml blood + 75 ml ACD solution), clamp the tube of blood donor set with an artery forcep to stop further flow of blood.
- Release the pressure in the arm to 0 mm Hg.
- Put a dry gauze piece over the needle and take it out of the donor's arm.
- Put a cotton swab over the site of puncture and advise the donor to hold it tightly with the help of other hand to stop the bleeding.
- Take the collecting set out of bottle and store away the bottle after collecting blood sample in two pilot tubes for test. Blood is stored in refrigerator at 4°C to 8°C.
- Put adhesive tape over the site of punctured vein after the bleeding stops.

Cross-matching of Blood

- It is must before issuing blood finally for transfusion to the patient.
- It must be done even if blood of donor and blood of patient is of same blood group.
- It is ordinarily done as under:
    - Take one clean slide and divide into two with a wax pencil. Mark them as 1 and 2.
    - Patients cell suspension, donor's serum and normal saline (one drop each) are taken on part of slide marked 1.

- Blood donor's cell suspension, patient's serum and normal saline (one drop each) are taken on the part of slide marked 2.
 - Rock the slide occasionally but gently for 5 minutes.
 - Now examine them under microscope for clumping. However, final examination under microscope is done after 15 minutes.
- Clumping or agglutination means blood cannot be transfused as it is incompatible.
- In general, remember that blood group 'O' person is universal donor (can give blood to a person of any group) while group AB is called universal recipient (can have blood of any group). Now this concept is of no value.

Types of Blood Transfusion Reactions

- Hemolytic reactions producing chest pain, lumbar pain (backache), chills, falling blood pressure, jaundice and formation of small quantity of urine or formation of no urine.
- Pyrogenic reactions producing chills and fever.
- Allergenic reactions like rashes, urticarial eruptions, etc.
- Bacterial contamination through transfusion may cause low blood pressure, shock and no formation of urine.
- Circulatory overload resulting in acute heart failure and edema of lungs.

SECTION 6

Histopathology

Section Outline
- ❖ Histopathology

CHAPTER 7

Histopathology

Histopathological Examination

The processing of piece of tissue (biopsy) is described below:

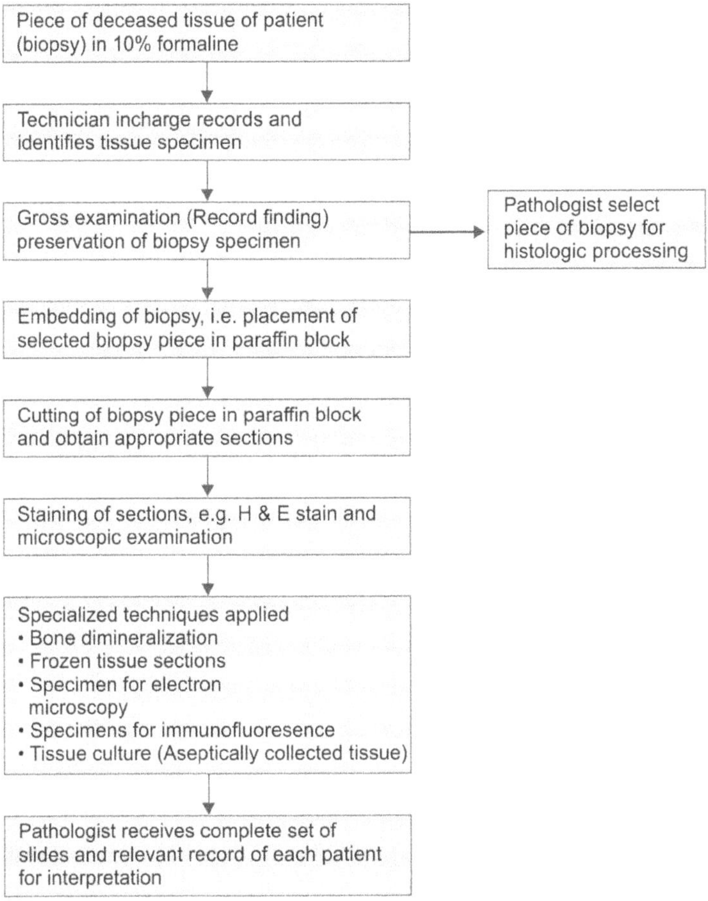

```
┌─────────────────────────────────────┐
│ Piece of deceased tissue of patient │
│ (biopsy) in 10% formaline           │
└─────────────────────────────────────┘
                │
                ▼
┌─────────────────────────────────────┐
│ Technician incharge records and     │
│ identifies tissue specimen          │
└─────────────────────────────────────┘
                │
                ▼
┌─────────────────────────────────────┐      ┌──────────────────────┐
│ Gross examination (Record finding)  │─────▶│ Pathologist select   │
│ preservation of biopsy specimen     │      │ piece of biopsy for  │
└─────────────────────────────────────┘      │ histologic processing│
                │                            └──────────────────────┘
                ▼
┌─────────────────────────────────────┐
│ Embedding of biopsy, i.e. placement │
│ of selected biopsy piece in paraffin│
│ block                               │
└─────────────────────────────────────┘
                │
                ▼
┌─────────────────────────────────────┐
│ Cutting of biopsy piece in paraffin │
│ block and obtain appropriate sections│
└─────────────────────────────────────┘
                │
                ▼
┌─────────────────────────────────────┐
│ Staining of sections, e.g. H & E    │
│ stain and microscopic examination   │
└─────────────────────────────────────┘
                │
                ▼
┌─────────────────────────────────────┐
│ Specialized techniques applied      │
│  • Bone dimineralization            │
│  • Frozen tissue sections           │
│  • Specimen for electron microscopy │
│  • Specimens for immunofluoresence  │
│  • Tissue culture (Aseptically      │
│    collected tissue)                │
└─────────────────────────────────────┘
                │
                ▼
┌─────────────────────────────────────┐
│ Pathologist receives complete set of│
│ slides and relevant record of each  │
│ patient for interpretation          │
└─────────────────────────────────────┘
```

Histopathological Techniques

Reception of Specimen

- Technician posted at the reception must check the requisition form duly filled.
- If requisition form is incompletely filled, it may be brought to the notice of doctor posted in histopathology section who may contact the doctor dealing with this patient for missing information.

Registration

- All specimens received must be recorded on reception register, along with necessary details, i.e. name of patient, age, sex, OPD or MRD number, ward number, bed number, name of the clinician, clinical diagnosis and organ/piece sent.
- On arrival, each specimen is given a number followed by year of entry, e.g. 1/97. This specimen will carry this number all along.

Fixation of Specimen before Grossing

- Fixation is the process of killing and hardening.
- Specimen may be sent in 10% formalin. Minimum amount of fixative should be 6 to 10 times the volume of the specimen.
- Hollow viscera like the stomach and intestine must be opened along the antimesenteric border. They may be pinned on paraffin tray of cork boards with mucosal side up and fixed in 10% formalin in this state overnight.
- Types of fixatives are:
    - Formalin solution 10% (widely used)
    - Zenker fluid
    - Lugol solution
    - Absolute alcohol
    - Acetone
    - Formalin neutral.

Grossing of Specimens

- Specimen should be handled with gloves.
- Instrument, board should be thoroughly washed in running water after grossing each specimen.

- Gross description should be recorded with care as per format:
  - Number of pieces and name of the specimen (uterus, ovary, stomach, etc.)
  - Size of each in cm/mm
  - Appearance
  - Color
  - Contour
- Blocks of lesional areas of specimen are cut for processing. Blocks should be thin (less than 4 mm) and trimmed to small size.
- Nearly every bone specimen requires some decalcification. Fragments of bone to demonstrate lesion, 3 mm thick sections is sawed from specimen for decalcification.
- Decalcification takes place using any of the following solutions:
  - 5% solution of nitric acid and hypochloric acid solution.
  - Formic acid sodium citrate solution.
  - Electrolytic method is used for decalcification. Electrolytic apparatus is used in formic acid hydrochloric acid for 1 to 4 hours. Then wash in running water for 24 hours. Now dehydrate it and embed it.

Labeling of Tissues

- After tissue is selected for processing, it is labeled with a number. This label bearing number of specimen through all stages of processing including section preparation and tissue blocks.
- Remains of all specimens are preserved in formalin until reported. Do not forget to write clearly number allotted to specimen.

Processing of Tissue Specimen

Dehydration

- After fixation, tissue is dehydrated by alcohol.
- Tissue is placed in 70% alcohol for 3 to 12 hours and then in 80%, 90% and 100% alcohol for 1, 2 and 3 hours.
- Amount of alcohol should be 10 to 20 times more than the tissue.
- After dehydration alcohol should be removed from tissue by clearing agent. Chloroform is commonly used for this purpose. Tissue is placed in pure chloroform for 4 to 8 hours.
- Now tissue is transferred to a mixture of equal parts of chloroform and paraffin for 4 to 8 hours.

Section 6: Histopathology

Impregnation with Paraffin Wax

- For routine work, paraffin wax is used having melting point 60°C.
- If tissue is less than 3 mm, it is kept in wax bath for 1 hour. In case tissue is 3 to 5 mm thick, it is kept in paraffin bath for 1 to 3 hours and require to be changed twice. And 5 to 10 mm thick tissue is placed in wax bath for 3 to 6 hours and is changed twice (**Fig. 7.1**).

Manual Processing Schedule

Formalin 10%	overnight	
Alcohol 80%		9 am to 11 am
Alcohol 90%		11 am to 1 pm
Absolute alcohol		1 pm to 4 pm
Absolute alcohol	overnight	
Chloroform		9 am to 11 am
Chloroform		11 am to 1 pm
Paraffin		1 pm to 3 pm
Paraffin		3 pm to 4 pm
Solidify	overnight	
Warm and the vacuum		9 am to 11 am embed and cool quickly

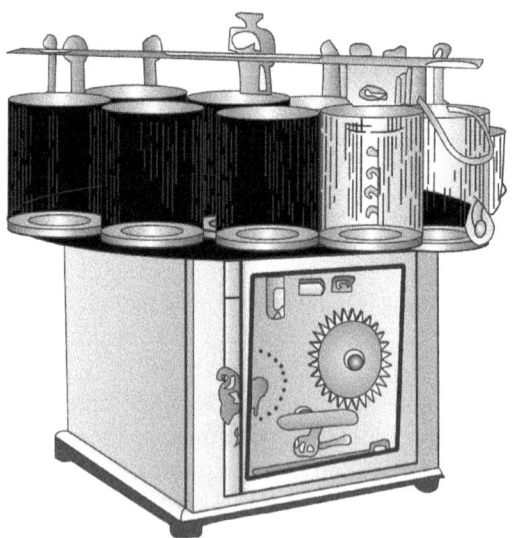

Fig. 7.1: An automatic tissue processing unit

Embedding of Tissue Specimen

- Embedding means, tissue is kept in molten paraffin.
- It provides a firm medium for keeping intact all parts of the tissue when cut.
- For this purpose mould used in the production of wax block are in leuk hart's, lead L's.
- Molten wax is put into the mould to a depth more than adequate to cover the thickest tissue block. When a thin film of semisolid wax has formed on the base of mould, the tissue with warmed forceps is kept into semisolid wax correctly.
- Now, dip it in cold water to solidify the wax quickly.

Cutting of Section

- It is done with the help of microtome (**Fig. 7.2**).
- Set microtome to cut section 5 to 10 micron in thickness.
- Cool the knife with ice. Set this cooled knife. Attach the block with pivot in microtome.
- Tighten all the screws and set the knife at the required angle.
- Adjust the block in such a way that the long side of tissue is parallel to knife edge.

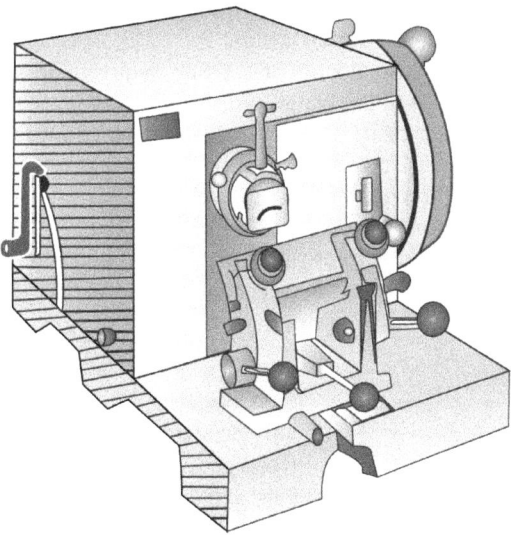

Fig. 7.2: Microtome

- Bring the block to knife by making appropriate adjustment of microtome.
- Now start cutting the tissue.
- Put the ribbons of sections on the surface of a large dish of warm water (45°C). Try to stretch the ribbon gently to remove wrinkles.

Mounting the Tissue on Slide

- Smear a clean slide with Mayer's albumin solution (egg white + glycerine + 1% sodium salicylate) and heat the slide slightly.
- Dip the slide under a section, place it in position on one side and lift the slide from water.
- Drain the excess water and pass the slide over spirit lamp. Keep the slide in slanting position for sometime to dry it.
- Keep slide in a box and keep it at 60°C for 1 hour.
- Keep the slide at room temperature before staining.
- This slide must bear the number allotted to specimen on its arrival.

Staining Procedure

- Place slides in xylol for 5 minutes, 3 minutes each in absolute alcohol in 95% alcohol in 80% alcohol and in 70% alcohol.
- Wash the slide in water for 5 minutes and rinse in distilled water.
- Stain in hematoxylin for 10 to 15 minutes.
- Rinse in water until section is blue.
- Treat it with 1% acid alcohol until tissue begins to appear.
- Wash the section in tap water.
- Now place the slide in ammonia water until section is again blue. It may require 3 to 5 dips.
- Wash in running water for 10 to 20 minutes.
- Stain in eosin for 15 seconds to 2 minutes.
- Dehydrate in 95% absolute alcohol until excess eosin is removed.
- Clear in xylol and mount the section with coverslip using DPX solution.

Results

Nuclei	Blue black
Cytoplasm	Varying shade of pink
Muscle fibers	Deep pinky red
Collagen	Pale pinky red
Red blood corpuscles	Orange to red
Fibrin	Deep pink

Museum Techniques

These are meant for pathology museum which has following uses:
- Permanent preservation of specimen showing diseased changes in organ.
- Collection of rare and interesting specimens.

Reception of Specimen
- Specimen from operation theaters, postmortem rooms and histopathology laboratories are sent.
- Permanent number along with relevant description should be printed on a tag attached or kept with specimen.

Preparation of Specimen
- Specimen should be fresh and without any preservative, when it is received.
- Gross trimming and dissection should be done to show the diseased part of the organ as clearly as possible.
- The specimen should be washed in normal saline only and not in water.
- Specimen may be photographed in their natural color before fixation.
- Solid organ can be sliced and placed flat on paraffin trays or cork boards and covered with cotton soaked in a formalin-based fixative.
- Cystic or hollow organs should be stuffed with cotton soaked in formalin to preserve their natural shape.
- Segments of intestine may be opened along antimesenteric edge and placed flat on paraffin trays or pinned on cork board and covered with cotton soaked in formalin.

Fixation of the Specimen
- All containers should be lined by fixative soaked lint or unfixed area may remain at points where specimen is in contact with the bottom of container.
- Perfusion through arteries may be done to fix solid organ, limbs, brain and heart.
- Fixative used has pH 7 and has following contents:

Formalin	1 liter
Potassium acetate	85 gm
Potassium nitrate	45 gm
Water	To make 10 liters

Restoration of Specimen

- The specimen is removed from fixative and washed in running water.
- It is transferred to 95% alcohol and kept as such for ½ hour to 12 hours.
- When natural color restoration is achieved, it is removed and placed in the preserving or mounting solution.

Preservation of Specimen

- Final preserving solution (K-3 solution) consists of:
  Sodium acetate   1416 gm
  Glycerine   4 liters
  Water to make   10 liters
- The specimen remains in this solution, until it is well permeated.

Presentation of Specimen

- Specimens may be mounted in glass jars available in many sizes.
- To support the specimen within the jar, it is attached to the specimen plate or a frame made of glass rods by tying or stitching after adjusting the specimen in its correct anatomical position.
- The container is filled with K-3 solution to the top to remove excess of air.
- The jar is closed with lid. Lid is properly sealed with jar using adhesives, e.g. araldite or fevicol.

Organization of Museum Specimens

- Each specimen bear code letter and number which is painted on the jar.
- Simple loose leaf catalog or files containing all necessary information regarding the specimen should be available for each and ready reference.

Fine Needle Aspiration Cytology

Fine needle aspiration cytology also called FNAC has become very popular diagnostic tool now-a-days. It is very simple, easy to perform, less time consuming, giving very less discomfort to patients, comparatively cheap and providing quick and reasonably accurate diagnosis.
Fine needle aspiration cytology is useful as under :
- May differentiate benign tumor from malignant tumor
- May help to classify tumors and other pathological processes

Uses of FNAC

- FNAC can be done on any patient
- This technique causes only slight discomfort
- This procedure does not carry major side effects

However, there is one caution that FNAC should not be done in a person having clotting disorders.

Contraindications of FNAC

FNAC should not be done in following conditions:
- Carotid body tumor
- Pheochromocytoma
- Prostatitis
- Hydatid cyst
- Pulmonary hypertension
- Severe hypoxemia
- Vascular lesions
- Ovarian cyst

Preparation of the Patient

- Explain the procedure and possible side effects to the patient
- Take informal consent of the patient
- No local anesthesia is required
- The skin is cleaned with alcohol at and around the area of operation
- In deep-seated tumors, larger area of skin is cleaned. Here use sterile gloves and draping must be made.

Aspiration Technique

Essentially, it requires palpation of tumor, its immobilization, proper needle-tip placements and movements. In fact aspiration is done as under:
- The tumor mass is fixed with one hand and with other hand aspiration is done
- Needle is inserted into the tumor mass and make to move to and fro 3 to 4 times in different directions
- Now the suction is applied by withdrawing the syringe plunger to 1 to 2 ml mark
- Optimal amount of tissue is collected in short time with minimum bleeding and discomfort

- After completion of aspiration, plunger is released before taking out the needle
- Now needle is disconnected and after filling the syringe with air, it is reconnected
- Now push the plunger quickly and expel the material onto the clean glass slide
- Tip of the needle should rest on the slide only to avoid any possible splattering

Side Effects and Complications of FNAC
- Local hematoma in and around the tumor mass
- Bleeding may occur during sampling
- Nerve paresis for short time
- Local infection
- Infarction of tumor
- Pneumothorax if tumor is near chest wall
- Tumor implantation

Smear Preparation

The basic idea of smear preparation is to allow optimal distribution of well-preserved small tissue pieces and cells on the clean glass slide. Smear is prepared by following two methods:

One-Step Method
- Two clean slides are held at right angles
- A small drop of aspirated material is placed near the frosted edge of the slide
- A second slide is then placed across the first one and moved downwards towards the material to cover the aspirated drop
- The smearing slide is moved quickly and smoothly with suitable pressure
- This smooth and gentle stroke gives optimal single layer smear for semisolid or small volume specimens.

Two-Step Particle Concentration and Smearing Method
- This method is useful for needle aspirates which are diluted by fluid
- A drop of aspirate is kept near the frosted end of grease-free and dust-free clean slide

- Bring the smearing slide onto the first slide at a point situated between drop of aspiration and observer
- Now smear is drawn by moving the sliding slide after touching the drop of aspiration
- This movement spreads much of the fluid over the central portion of stationary slide
- Most of the particles with small amount of fluid remain at the line of slide intersection
- This finishes the first step
- Sliding slide is placed over smeared slide and rotated slightly
- As soon as two slides come in contact, they are slowly and carefully pulled apart giving one-layered smear.

Staining of Aspirated Material

Papanicolaou's stain requires immediate fixation in alcohol before smear starts to dry. For purpose, ethanol (95%) is most commonly used.

Papanicolaou's Stain

Harris Hematoxylin

Hematoxylin	1 gm
Absolute alcohol	10 ml
Potassium alum	20 gm
Distilled water	200 ml
Mercuric oxide	0.5 gm

Preparation

- Hematoxylin is dissolved in absolute alcohol and potassium alum in distilled water with the help of heat
- The above two solutions are mixed together and boil for some time.
- Now mercuric oxide is added slowly but in very small quantity repeatedly
- The container containing the solution is immersed into cold water bath
- Allow the above solution to cool. After cooling, it is filtered and stored in a colored bottle.

Orange G6

Orange G	0.5 gm
95% ethyl alcohol	100 ml
Phosphotungstic acid	0.15 gm

Eosin Azure 36 (EA 36)

- Light green (SF) contains:
Light green (SF)	0.5 gm
95% ethyl alcohol	100 ml
- Eosin yellow contains:
Eosin yellow	0.5 gm
95% ethyl alcohol	100 ml

From the stock solution, the working solution of EA 36 is prepared as under:

Solution (1)	45 ml
Solution (2)	45 ml
Phosphotungstic acid	0.200 gm

All the above, solutions are stored in refrigerator.

Staining Procedure

The fixed slides are passed directly from fixative to the following solution as under:

80% ethyl alcohol	10 dips
70% ethyl alcohol	10 dips
50% ethyl alcohol	10 dips
Distilled water	3 min
Harris hematoxylin	1 min
Running tap water	1 min
Hydrochloric acid (0.5%)	5 dips
Running tap water	1 min
Dilute solution of lithium carbonate	1 min
Running tap water	1 min
50% ethyl alcohol	10 dips
70% ethyl alcohol	10 dips
80% ethyl alcohol	10 dips
95% ethyl alcohol	10 dips
Orange G6	1 min
95% ethyl alcohol	10 dips
EA 36	4 min
95% ethyl alcohol	10 dips
Absolute alcohol	4 min
Xylene	5 min

Slides may be mounted with DPX.

Results

Nucleus	Blue color
Cytoplasm of superficial cell	Pink color
Cytoplasm of intermediate cell	Bluish green color
Red blood cell	Orange

Rapid Staining Techniques

These methods are useful for preliminary study and evaluation of material. The methods are :
- Fast version of Papanicolaou's method
- H & E stain is actually meant for frozen sections
- Diff Quick—staining time is 2 minutes
- May-Grunwald-Giemsa staining time is 2 minutes
- Toluidine blue method is the fastest method (1 minute).

Toluidine Blue Method

- Immerse the smear in alcohol for at least 15 seconds
- 1 or 2 drops of toluidine blue solution (0.05 gm toluidine blue powder, 20 ml 95% alcohol and 80 ml distilled water mixed and filter before use) is applied to the smear
- Wet smear is mounted with coverslip
- Stain is allowed to penetrate for 10 to 15 seconds. Slide is turned over onto a towel or other absorbent material with coverslip in place and excess stain is removed after applying moderate pressure to the slide.
- The slide is ready for preliminary evaluation in about one minute
- After evaluation, the slide is immersed in alcohol. The coverslip will fall and now slide again is ready to stain by Papanicolaou method or by H & E method.
- The alcohol used above will also remove toluidine blue from cell
- If chosen to use May-Grunwald-Giemsa (Diff Quick), the stain will be less dense than applied otherwise.

Frozen Section

Tissue is frozen by keeping in ice. Sections are cut on freezing microtome.

Fixation

Usually biopsies for immediate diagnosis from operation theatre are cut without using any fixative. However, fixative of choice for frozen sections is 10% formalin saline. Small pieces of tissues are dipped in preheated 10% formalin for 10 to 20 minutes at 60°C.

After fixation following steps are undertaken:
- Tissue bits is treated with gum syrup for 1 to 5 minutes and transferred to the stage of a suitable freezing microtome of CO_2 cooling system.
- A filter paper soaked in water is kept on stage, coating of gum is applied with brush before the tissue is kept.
- With intermittent short exposure of CO_2 for 1 to 2 second and with pause of 3 to 4 seconds and the application of gum syrup or water, the tissue is frozen, well fixed on stage.
- 10 to 15 micron sections are cut by moving the knife lever.
- Sections are collected from knife blade with a wet brush into watch glass or small bowl containing water.
- Now the sections are stained by transferring them to watch glasses containing the required stain.
- Now they are dehydrated, cleared and mounted.
- Alternatively mounting may be done on clean glass slide coated with egg albumin glycerine mixture and stained as required.

Staining Technique for Rapid Diagnosis

- Place frozen sections on slide in 90% alcohol for 1 to 2 seconds.
- Transfer to absolute alcohol for 1 to 2 seconds.
- Transfer to xylol and agitate the slide until the section becomes clear (1 to 2 seconds).
- Transfer to absolute alcohol for 1 to 2 seconds.
- Transfer to 90% alcohol for 1 to 2 seconds.
- Stain with hematoxylin for 2 minutes.
- Rinse in tap water and dip in acid alcohol.
- Wash with tap water to which few drops of lithium carbonate have been already added.
- Leave the section in this solution for 20 to 30 seconds.
- Counterstain with 1% eosin for 10 to 15 seconds. Now rinse in water.
- Dehydrate successively with 90% alcohol and then with absolute alcohol.
- Clean with xylol in mount in DPX.

Exfoliative Cytology

It is a study of exfoliated cells collected as smears from different sites fixed in ethanol and stained by appropriate stains like papanicolaou stain. It may be sputum smear, cervical smear, vaginal smear, urine, CSF, gastric lavage, etc.

Uses
- Malignant cytology
- Hormonal cytology
- Screening for cervical cancer
- For sex chromatin
- Diagnosis of inflammation, dysplasia.

Special Staining Methods
Van Gieson's Stain
Requirement
Solution A
- Hematoxylin 1 gm
- Absolute alcohol 100 ml

Solution B
- 30% ferric chloride 4 ml
- Distilled water 95 ml
- Conc HCL 1 ml
    - Solution A and B are mixed before use.
    - 2 part of solution A and 1 part of solution B.

Procedure
- Bring section to water and stain for 3 minutes with Weigert's hematoxylin
- Wash in water for 5 minutes.
- Stain for 1 minute with piero-fuchsin (acid fuchsin 1%) solution 10 ml + 90 ml of saturated solution of pierce acid.
- Dehydrate, clear in xylol and mount it in acid balsam.

Result
- Collagen fibers = pink colored
- Other tissue = yellow colored

Stain for Amyloid

Procedure
- Bring sections to water and stain with 1% methyl violet for 5 to 10 minutes.
- Wash in water and differentiate in 1% acetic acid for few seconds and wash in water.
- Mount in glycerine jelly.

Result
Amyloid under artificial light = Purple pink

Stain for Hemosiderin (Perls Stain)

Procedure
- Bring section to water.
- Stain with a boiled mixture of equal parts.
- 2% potassium ferrocyanide and 2% HCL for 15 to 20 minutes.
- Wash it with water.
- Counterstain 1% aqueous eosin for few seconds.
- Wash, dehydrate and mount on DPX or Canada balsam.

Result
Iron pigment = Blue

Wilder's Silver Impregnation Method (Reticulum Fibers)

This method is especially useful to stain material fixed in formalin and embedded in paraffin.

Fixation
- Fix in 10% formalin, Zenker's or Helly fluid
- Embed it in paraffin and cut frozen sections
- Paraffin sections are mounted on slides before staining.

Staining Solution

- Ammoniacal silver hydroxide solution is prepared: To 5 ml of 10.2% aqueous solution of silver nitrate add 26 to 28 ammonium water drop by drop until the precipitates so formed get dissolved.
- Now make this solution upto 50 ml with distilled water.
- Reducing solution is prepared by taking 50 ml formalin neutralized with magnesium carbonate, 0.5 ml uranium nitrate and 1% aqueous solution 1.5 ml.

Staining Technique

- Sections are kept from water into 0.25% aqueous solution of potassium permanganate for one minute. Alternatively, 10% solution of phosphomolybdic acid may used.
- Rinse in distilled water.
- Place in 4% hydrobromic acid distilled water 1: 3 for one minute.
- Wash in tap water and then distilled water.
- Dip in 1% aqueous solution of uranium nitrate for 5 seconds only
- Wash with distilled water for 10 to 20 seconds
- Keep in ammoniacal silver solution for one minute
- Dip quickly in 95% alcohol
- Keep for one minute in reducing solution
- Wash in distilled water
- Tone in 1:500 aqueous gold chloride solution
- Rinse in distilled water
- Place in 5% aqueous solution of thiosulfate for 1 to 2 minute
- Wash in tap water
- Counterstain with alum hematoxylin and Van Gieson's stain
- Differentiate in 95% alcohol and dehydrate, clear in xylol. Now mount in Canada balsam

Result

- Fine reticulum fibers = Black color
- Collagen = Rose color

Staining for Fat

- Frozen sections from water are rinsed in 70% alcohol.

- Now it is transferred to staining solution, e.g. Sudan III for 10 to 15 minutes
- Differentiate it in 70% alcohol to remove excess of stain. Now rinse it in water.
- Stain in hematoxylin and differentiate rapidly in 1% aqueous HCL
- Mount it in glycerine jelly.

Verhoeff's Elastic Stain

- Stain section in staining solution for 15 minutes.
- Staining solution:
    - Solution A 5% hematoxylin in absolute alcohol
    - Solution B is 10% aqueous solution of ferric chloride
    - Solution C is:
        - Iodine 2 gm
        - Potassium iodide 4 gm
        - Distilled water 100 ml
- For use mix 10 parts of Solution A, 4 parts of solution B and 4 parts of solution C
- Differentiate in 2% ferric chloride, controlling differentiation with the microscope.
- Wash in water.
- Place it in 5% sodium thiosulfate for 1 minute to remove iodine. Now wash it with tap water for 5 minutes.
- Counterstain in Van Gieson's stain
- Differentiate, dehydrate, clear in xylol and mount

Result

- Elastic fiber = Black
- Nuclei = Blue to black
- Collagen = Red
- Other tissue = Yellow

SECTION 7

Biochemistry

DS Jamwal

Section Outline
- Biochemistry

Biochemistry

Introduction

As a matter of fact medical biochemistry (chemistry of life) deals with molecules of living cells and their chemical reactions. Medical laboratory technicians must understand and learn various laboratory techniques of biochemistry like estimation in serum/blood of sugar, urea, cholesterol, uric acid, proteins and many others. The normal values of above are known. In diseases, these normal values either become more or less than normal. Blood for tests should be collected when patient is on fast for 8 to 12 hours.

Estimation of Blood Glucose

Glucose is present in the blood and is used by different body tissues for energy. Tissues like brain utilize only glucose to meet its need of energy. The source of blood glucose is food carbohydrates. Food carbohydrates are digested to glucose or converted to glucose. During the interval between meals blood glucose is maintained by liver glycogen.

Ortho-toluidine Method

Principle

Glucose in serum reacts with o-toluidine (in glacial acetic acid) at 100°C to form, N-glycosyl amine, a blue-green condensation product, which absorbs maximum light in the red wavelength at 600–630 nm.

Reagents

- *Ortho-toluidine reagent*: To 470 ml glacial acetic acid (AR) add 0.75 gm thiourea. Shake to dissolve thiourea and add 30 ml o-toluidine (AR). Mix by repeated inversion and transfer to amber-colored reagent bottles. Use after standing overnight. Store at room temperature.
- *Stock glucose solution 1 gm%*: Dissolve 1 gm AR grade dry glucose powder in about 70 to 80 ml 0.1% benzoic acid in a 100 ml volumetric

flask and make the volume to 100 ml with benzoic acid (keep at 2–8°C).
- *Working standards 100 mg%*: Transfer 10.0 ml, stock glucose standard to a 100 ml volumetric flask and dilute to the volume with 0.1% benzoic acid (keep at 2–8°C).

Procedure

Label test tubes (100 × 12 mm) as 'B' (blank), 'S' (standard), 'T' (test) and pipette into the tubes as follows:

	B	S	T
Distilled water	50 µl	–	–
Standard (100 mg%)	–	50 µl	–
Plasma/serum	–	–	50 µl
o-toluidine reagent	3.0 ml	3.0 ml	3.0 ml

Mix the contents and keep the tubes simultaneously in a boiling water bath and allow to boil for 10 minutes. Remove the tubes from the water bath and cool to room temperature in water. Set the colorimeter/spectrophotometer to zero optical density (OD) with blank using red filter or a wavelength of 630 nm and read OD of standard and tests.

Precaution

o-toluidine reagent is corrosive so do not pipette with mouth and avoid contact with skin and eyes.

Calculations

Concentration of glucose, mg/100 ml = OD of test/OD of standard × 100

$$mg/dl = \frac{OD \text{ of Test}}{OD \text{ of Standard}} \times 200$$

Normal Values

Normal fasting serum/plasma glucose in healthy adults = 65 mg–110/mg/dl. After meals, the level goes up and may reach upto 170 mg/dl and comes down to fasting level within 2 hours.

Interpretation

Blood sugar level is raised in diabetes mellitus. Some rise is also seen in pancreatic diseases, infections diseases, intracranial diseases over activity of thyroid, pituitary and adrenal glands and after anesthesia. Low blood glucose levels are found after insulin overdose, in low activity of thyroid, adrenal, pituitary glands and glycogen storage disease.

The true blood glucose level is estimated by glucose oxidase method. The o-toluidine gives values near to true blood sugar. Other methods estimate 15 to 20% higher than true blood sugar. Plasma/serum sugar values are 10 to 15% higher than whole blood, due to difference in water concentrate.

Other Methods for Estimation of Blood Glucose Levels

Enzymatic Method

It is based on the action of enzyme glucose-oxidase on glucose to form gluconic acid and hydrogen peroxide. Oxygen formed from hydrogen peroxide in presence of peroxidase, oxidizes phenol which gives red color with 4-amino antipyrine.

Ferricyanide Method

In this method, ferricyanide in alkaline solution is reduced to ferrocyanide. The amount of ferrocyanide is measured by many ways.

Methods which utilize reduction of alkaline copper sulfate Folin-Wu, Nelson Somogyi, etc.

Principle

A protein-free blood filtrate is treated with alkaline copper solution, the cuprous oxide formed is treated with a phosphomolybdic acid solution, blue color being obtained which is compared with that of standard.

Requirements

- Alkaline $CuSO_4$ solution.
- Phosphomolybdate acid solution.
- Standard glucose solution (0.1 mg/ml)
- Sodium tungstate solution 10% 2/3N H_2SO_4.

Procedure

	B	S	T
Distilled water	3.2 ml	3.2 ml	3.2 ml
Blood	–	–	0.2 ml
Standard	–	0.2 ml	–
Distilled water	0.2 ml	–	–
Sodium tungstate 10%	0.3 ml	0.3 ml	0.3 ml
2/3 N H_2SO_4	0.2 ml	0.3 ml	0.3 ml
Mix well and centrifuge at 3000 rpm for 3 minutes			
Clear filtrate from above	2.0 ml	2.0 ml	2.0 ml
Alkaline copper reagent	2.0 ml	2.0 ml	2.0 ml
Mix and keep in boiling water for 10 minutes			

Cool for 2 to 3 minutes and add 2 ml phosphomolybdic acid to each tube and dilute 25 ml with distilled water. Read in colorimeter, using red filter and setting zero OD with distilled water.

Calculation

$$\text{Blood sugar (mg/dl)} = \frac{\text{OD test} - \text{OD blank}}{\text{OD Std} - \text{OD blank}} \times 200$$

Interpretation

- Normal fasting venous blood sugar values are 80 to 120 mg/dl.
- Fasting hyperglycemia is suggestive of diabetes mellitus.

Glucose Tolerance Test (GTT)

Preparation of Patients

- Patient should be ambulatory and free from stress for about 2 weeks before test.
- Patient should be on liberal carbohydrate diet for at least 3 to 4 days before the test.
- Collect fasting venous blood and urine sample.
- Give 50 to 100 gm of glucose in 300 to 400 ml water by mouth and note the exact timing.

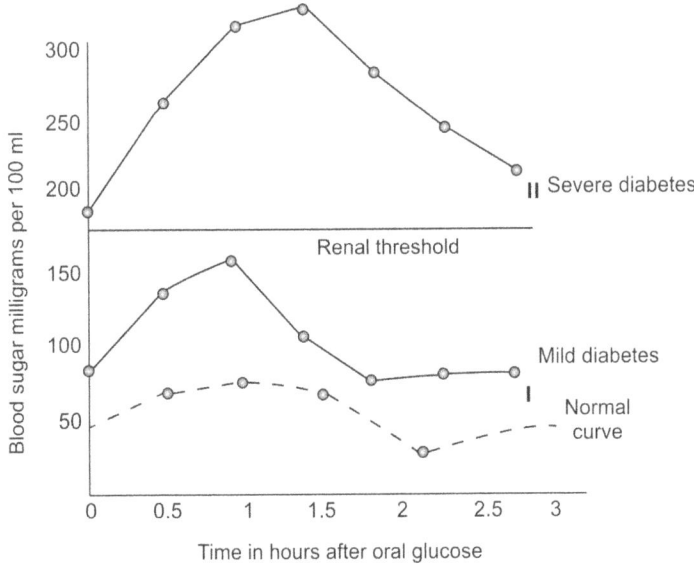

Fig. 8.1: Glucose tolerance test curve

- Further blood and urine samples are taken at 30, 60, 90 and 120 minutes.
- Test each blood sample as discussed in blood sugar estimation and urine samples for the presence of sugar.
- Plot GTT curve **(Fig. 8.1)**.

Normal Values

Fasting value   60 to 100 mg/dl
One hour value   120 to 150 mg/dl
Two hours value   back to fasting
No glycosuria is observed in any sample.

Diabetic Curve

- GTT curve is raised and prolonged
- Glycosuria is seen.

Renal Glycosuria

- The curve is normal.
- One or more samples of urine contain glucose.

Lag Stage Curve

- Fasting value normal.
- Maximum value at 30 minutes is >180 mg/dl with glycosuria.

Flat Curve of Enhanced GT

- Fasting value is < normal and throughout the test level does not vary by more than ± 20 mg/dl.

Diagnostic Glucose Values for Oral GTT

Conditions	Fasting	2 hours postprandial
Diabetes mellitus	>120 mg/dl	>180 mg/dl
Impaired GTT	>120 mg/dl	120–180 mg/dl
Normal	>100 mg/dl	<120 mg/dl

Blood Urea Estimation

Urea, a nitrogenous compound is formed in the body in liver. It is formed from ammonia formed during catabolism of amino acids, the building blocks of proteins. It is an end product of protein metabolism. It is water soluble and is excreted through urine. In normal adults, 30 to 35 gm urea is excreted in urine in 24 hours.

Diacetyl Monoxime (DAM) Method

Principle

Urea present in serum/plasma reacts directly with diacetyl monoxime in presence of Fe^{3+} ions and thiosemicarbazide at 100°C to form red colored soluble complex in acidic medium which is measured at blue-green wavelength (520 to 540 nm).

Reagents

- *Acid reagent stock A*: Ferric chloride ($FeCl_3.6H_2O$) 2 gm + 10 ml distilled water. Dissolve and add 40 ml phosphoric acid and slowly add water to make 100 ml.
- *Acid reagent stock B*: Conc. H_2SO_4 200 ml + DW 800 ml
- *Working acid reagent* Acid reagent A 0.5 ml + Acid reagent B 1000 ml.

- *Color reagent stock A*: Diacetyl monoxime, 2% in water.
- *Color reagent stock B*: Thiosemicarbazide 0.5% in water.
- *Working color reagent* Stock color reagent A and B 67 ml each and water to 1000 ml.
- *Stock urea standard* prepare 1 gm% urea in phenylmercuric acetate (4 mg% phenylmercuric acetate containing a drop of H_2SO_4).
- *Working standard* Dilute 3 ml of stock to 100 ml with phenylmercuric acetate.

Procedure

Label two test tubes (18 × 150 mm) as T (test) S (standard)

	Test	Standard
Add water	10 ml	10 ml
Plasma/serum	0.1 ml	–
Standard (working)	–	0.1 ml

Mix by repeated inversions.
Prepare another set of test tubes T (test) S (standard) and B (blank).

	T	S	B
Add water	1.0 ml	1.0 ml	2.0 ml
Diluted serum from above	1.0 ml	–	–
Diluted standard from above	–	1.0 ml	–
Working color reagent	2.0 ml	2.0 ml	2.0 ml
Working acid reagent	2.0 ml	2.0 ml	2.0 ml

Mix thoroughly and place the tube simultaneously in boiling water bath for 20 minutes. Cool the tubes and take OD at green filter at a wavelength of 520 to 540 nm. Setting zero OD with distilled water.

Calculation

$$\text{Serum/plasma urea mg\%} = \frac{T - B}{S - B} \times 40$$

Normal Value

15 to 45 mg%

Interpretation

Raised in prerenal causes (prolonged vomiting, excessive diarrhea hematemesis).

Renal cause: All forms of kidney diseases.

Postrenal causes: Enlargement of prostrate, stones in the urinary tract, tumor of bladder, stricture of urethera.

Other Methods

Urease Method

In most of the techniques, the conversion of urea to ammonium carbonate by an enzyme urease present in jackbeans and soybeans is used for quantitive estimation. The ammonium ion formed is then measured colorimetrically by nesslerization or by Berthelot reaction with phenol and hypochlorite.

Blood Creatinine Estimation

Alkaline Picrate Method

Creatinine is derived from creatine and is a waste product. It is largely endogenous in origin, unless the diet is rich in meat.

Principle

Creatinine reacts with picric acid in presence of NaOH to form a red colored complex (Jaffe's reaction). The color appears in different shades of orange, due to yellow color of picric acid and creatinine concentration.

Reagents

- *Picric acid*: Prepare saturated solution of picric acid at room temperature.
- *Sodium hydroxide 0.75 N. 3%*: Weigh quickly 30 gm of NaOH, dissolve in water and dilute to 1000 ml.
- *Standard creatinine stock*: 100 mg% dissolve 100 mg of accurately weighed creatinine powder in 0.1NHCl and dilute to 100 ml with the same acid.

- Working creatinine standard (2 mg%): Dilute 2 ml of stock standard to 100 ml with water.
- Sodium tungstate 5%
- Sulfuric acid 2/3N

Procedure

Label 12 × 100 ml test tubes as B (blank) S (standard) and T (tests) and add as follows:

	B	S	T
Serum	–	–	0.5 ml
Stand (2 mg%)	–	0.5 ml	–
Water	4.0 ml	3.5 ml	3.5 ml
5% sodium tungstate	0.5 ml	0.5 ml	0.5 ml
2/3N H_2SO_4	0.5 ml	0.5 ml	0.5 ml

Shake and centrifuge at 2500 to 3000 rpm ater 8 to 10 minutes. To another set of 18 × 150 mm test tubes labeled as earlier.

	B	S	T
Supernatant from earlier	3.0 ml	3.0 ml	3.0 ml
Picric acid solution	1.0 ml	1.0 ml	1.0 ml
Sodium hydroxide (0.75N)	1.0 ml	1.0 ml	1.0 ml

Keep at a fixed temperature between (25–37%) for 15 min. Read OD at 520 to 540 nm wavelength or using green filter adjusting zero with DW.

Calculation

Creatinine mg/dl = OD Test – OD Blank/OD Standard – OD Blank × 2

Normal Values

0.9 to 1.5 mg/dl in males
0.7 to 1.3 mg/dl in females

Interpretation

Values above normal are seen in renal disease, when it rises somewhat parallel to serum urea. Small rise is seen in intestinal obstruction or heart failures.

Low values are found in muscle dystrophy.

Other methods: Various methods used are mostly the modification utilizing the Jaffe's reaction.

Estimation of Total Proteins and Albumin in Blood

Biuret Method for Total Protein

Proteins

Proteins in plasma are divided into three types: Albumin, globulins and Fibrinogen. Serum contains no fibrinogen. The plasma/serum proteins are altered in various pathological conditions and their estimation is useful for diagnosis and follow-up.

Principle

A violet-colored chelation complex is formed between peptide linkages of amino acids in proteins and copper ions in alkaline medium.

Reagents

- *Biuret reagent*: Dissolve 3 gm of copper sulfate in about 500 ml of 0.1N NaOH. Add 9 gm of sodium-potassium tartarate and 5 gm of potassium iodide. Dissolve and dilute the contents to 1000 ml (store at room temperature).
- *Biuret blank*: Prepare the above solution without copper sulfate.
- *Normal saline with sodium azide:* NaCl 9 gm + sodium azide 1 gm, dissolve and make up to 1 liter.
- Prepare a standard of 7.0 gm/dl from dry bovine serum albumin in normal saline—sodium azide solution or use a non-hemolyzed, non-jaundiced clear serum whose protein concentration is already measured.

  Label 15 × 150 nm test tubes as B (blank), S (standard) and T (tests 1, 2, 3, etc.) and pipette into the tubes as follows:

	B	S	T	(TB)*
Biuret reagent (ml)	2.5	2.5	2.5	–
Distilled water (µl)	50	–	–	–
Protein standard (7gm% (µl)	–	50	–	–
Serum sample (µl)	–	–	50	50
Biuret blank (ml)	–	–	–	2.5

*In case of turbid samples prepare a "Test blank" tube.

Mix well and keep at 37°C for 10 minutes or 25°C for 30 minutes. Take the OD with yellow green filter or at 540 nm setting zero with blank.

Calculation

$$\text{Serum protein (gm/dl)} = \frac{\text{OD of Test}}{\text{OD of Std}} \times 7 \text{ (or Conc. of serum standard)}$$

Normal Values

Total proteins/dl
Adults 6.5–8.5 gm/dl
Children 5.4–8.7 gm/dl
Neonates 5.2–9.1 gm/dl

Interpretation

- Increased in (i) dehydration, (ii) multiple myeloma, and (iii) hyperglobulinemia.
- Decreased in (i) nephrotic syndrome; (ii) proteinuria; (iii) burns; (iv) exudative dermatosis; (v) idiopathic exudative enteropathy; and (vi) enteritis, colitis, fistulae, amyloidosis, lymph node metastasis, etc.

Albumin

BCG Method

(Bartholomew and Delaney, 1966)

Principle

Albumin in serum or plasma when treated with buffered BCG at a pH acidic to its isoelectric pH, binds the dye to form a greenish complex, the intensity of the color is proportional to the concentration of albumin.

Reagents

- *Bromocresol green solution*: To about 900 ml of DW, add in the following order and dissolve, succinic acid 5.6 gm, bromocresol green (Na salt) 58 mg, sodium azide 100 mg, sodium hydroxide

1.0 gm. Brij-35 solution 2.5 ml. Adjust to pH 4.2 with 5% succinic acid or 0.5N NaOH. Dilute to 1 liter (Stable for several months at 2 to 8°C).
- *Succinate Buffer*: Prepare exactly as solution number-1 without adding the dye.
- Prepare a 5 gm/dl solution of bovine serum albumin in normal saline containing 100 mg/dl sodium azide.

Procedure

Label 15 × 150 mm test tubes as B (blank) S (standard) and T (test 1, 2, etc.) and pipette into the tubes as follows:

	B	S	T
BCG solution (ml)	4.0	4.0	4.0
Water (μl)	20	–	–
Albumin standard 5 gm% (μl)	–	20	–
Serum sample (μl)	–	–	20

Mix the blank tube well and adjust the colorimeter, spectrophotometer to zero with the blank with red filter or a wavelength of 632 nm. Prepare the S tube and immediately take OD. Mix the test tube T1 take reading and so on (reading should be taken within 30 seconds of mixing sample with the dye).

Note: In case of turbid lipemic sample, prepare a serum blank tube adding 4.0 ml of succinate buffer instead of dye.

Calculation

$$\text{Serum albumin (gm/dl)} = \frac{\text{OD Test}}{\text{OD Std}} \times 5$$

Normal Values

3.5 to 5.5 gm/dl

Interpretation

- Raised in dehydration
- Decreased in kidney diseases, GI tract disorders, burns, malnutrition, liver disorders.

Other Methods

- In Kjeldahl nesslerization method, proteins are digested with sulphuric acid and the nitrogen converted to ammonium sulfate Ammonium sulfate reacts with Nessler's reagent to a yellow-colored compound
- Rough estimation can be done by specific gravity method
- Albumin can be separated by ammonium sulfate precipitation of globulins and then estimated by Biuret method
- Separation of various globulins can be accomplished by electrophoresis.

Blood Cholesterol Estimation

Cholesterol (a lipid) is both of endogenous and dietary origin. Its raised values may lead to serious ailments.

Ferric Chloride Method of Henley

Principle

Cholesterol is oxidized by ferric ions and disulfuric acid. The oxidized products polymerize and combine with disulfuric acid to form a purple Colored sulfonated polymer. The color is proportional to the cholesterol concentration in the original sample.

Reagents

- Aldehyde-free glacial acetic acid (AR/GR)
- Concentrated sulfuric acid (AR/GR)
- Ferric chloride ($FeCl_3.6H_2O$) 0.05% in glacial acetic acid.

Cholesterol standard 200 mg/dl in glacial acetic acid.

Procedure

Prepare a set of clean dry test tubes 18 × 150 mm. Pipette into the tubes:

	T	S	B
Serum (µl)	100	–	–
Standard 200 mg/dl (µl)	–	100	–
Water (µl)	–	–	100
Ferric chloride (reagent 3) (ml)	5 ml	5 ml	5 ml

Allow to stand at room temperature for 30 minutes and centrifuge.

	T	S	B
Supernatant from the above step into another set of tubes (ml)	5	5	5
Sulfuric acid [reagent (2) ml]	3	3	3

Mix thoroughly by pouring into a clean dry test tube and stand till the tubes are cooled to room temperature (20 to 30 minutes)

Read at 580 nm or orange filter (in case orange filter is not available yellow green filter can be used). Use water for adjusting zero.

Calculation

$$\text{Serum cholesterol mg/dl} = \frac{\text{OD Test} - \text{OD Blank}}{\text{OD Std} - \text{OD Blank}} \times 250$$

Normal Values

130 to 250 mg% (increase with age)

Interpretation

- Raised values seen in diabetes mellitus hypothyroidism obstructive jaundice, essential hypercholesterolemia, essential hyperlipidemia, pregnancy, high fatty diet.
- Lowered valued are often seen in malnutrition, hyperthyroidism, severe hepatic damage.

Other Methods

- Using Liebermann-Burchard reaction
- Enzymatic methods are based on the following sequence of reaction:

$$\text{Cholesterol esters} \xrightarrow{\text{Cholesterol esterase}} \text{Cholesterol + fatty acids}$$

$$\text{Cholesterol esters} \xrightarrow{\text{Cholesterol oxidase}} \text{Cholet-4en-3-one} + H_2O_2$$

$$H_2O_2 + \text{Phenol} + \text{4-aminoantipyrine} \xrightarrow{\text{Peroxidase}} \text{Red quinone} + H_2O$$

Serum Bilirubin

Bilirubin is an end product of hemoglobin breakdown. It is excreted by liver through bile as a conjugated product. In normal serum, it is mainly present in the unconjugated form. Conjugated form is found in diseased state.

Method of Malloy and Evelyn

Principle

The method is based on the formation of a purple-colored compound azobilirubin, when bilirubin reacts with diazotized sulfanilic acid (diazo reagent) introduced by Van den Bergh. Methanol is added in an amount insufficient to precipitate proteins yet sufficient to permit all bilirubin to react with diazo reagent.

Reagents

Diazo 'A' 1 gm sulfanilic acid in 1.5% HCl/L.
Diazo 'B' 0.5 gm. sodium nitrite/100 ml in water.
Diazo reagent: Prepare freshly by mixing 0.3 ml Diazo 'B' with 10 ml Diazo 'A'.
Diazo blank: HCl 1.5% in water.

Absolute Methanol:
Bilirubin standard (10 mg/dl) Prepare a solution of pure bilirubin powder 10 mg in 100 ml chloroform. Try to dissolve the powder completely by refluxing the mixture gently.

Procedure

Label a set of 15 × 150 mm test tubes as Tt (test total) Tb (test blank), Tc (Test conjugated) Tcb (test conjugated blank), St (standard), Stb (standard blank) and add as follows:

	Tt	Tb	Tc	Tcb	St	Stb
Distilled water (ml)	0.8	0.8	0.8	0.8	–	–
Absolute methanol (ml)	–	–	–	–	1.8	1.8
Serum (ml)	0.2	0.2	0.2	0.2	–	–
Standard 10 mg/dl (ml)	–	–	–	–	0.2	0.2
Diazo reagent (ml)	0.5	–	0.5	–	0.5	0.5
Diazo blank (ml)	–	0.5	–	0.5	–	0.5
Methanol (ml)	2.5	2.5	–	–	2.5	2.5
Water (ml)	–	–	2.5	2.5	–	–

Mix the contents and keep for 3.0 minutes at room temperature, preferably in dark.

Take the OD with yellow green filter or at a wavelength of 540 nm, using water for zero setting.

Calculation

$$\text{Serum bilirubin total mg/dl} = \frac{\text{OD Test} - \text{OD Tb}}{\text{OD St} - \text{OD St B}} \times 10$$

Serum bilirubin conjugated (mg/dl) =

$$\frac{\text{OD Test conjugated} - \text{OD Test conjugated blank}}{\text{OD St} - \text{OD Std blank}} \times 10 \times 1.05$$

Note: Conjugated bilirubin shows a lower OD in water, hence to be multiplied by a factor of 1.05

Normal Values

Total bilirubin 0.5 to 1.2 mg/dl
Conjugated bilirubin 0.0 to 0.6 mg/dl

Interpretations

Elevated values of:
- Conjugated bilirubin are found in posthepatic obstruction, intrahepatic cholestasis, acute hepatitis, liver dystrophy, liver cirrhosis.
- Unconjugated bilirubin are found in hemolytic jaundice, neonatal jaundice, hemoglobinopathies, liver disease, malaria incompatible blood transfusions due to drugs such as primaquine in G6PD deficient subjects.

Other methods are modified using Van den Bergh reaction
Bilirubin can also be estimated by reading the absorption of bilirubin at various wavelengths such as 454 and 575 nm.

Estimation of Serum Uric Acid

Caraway Methods

Uric acid is an end product of purine metabolism and is excreted through urine.

Principle

Phosphotungstic acid is reduced by uric acid in the presence of sodium carbonate to give a blue complex which absorbs light at 710 nm or red light.

Reagents

- *Sodium tungstate* 10% w/v in water.
- *2/3 N sulfuric acid* 18 ml of conc. sulfuric acid, mixed with water and made to 1000 ml with water.
- *Sodium carbonate* 14 gm of anhydrous Na_2CO_3 per 100 ml in water.
- *Phosphotungstate reagent* (Readymade commercially available or prepared) 50 mg sodium tungstate + 400 ml water + 40 ml phosphoric acid (85%). Reflux gently for 2 hours. Cool and make the volume to 500 ml store in brown bottle. Dilute 1:10 before use.
- *Uric acid standard* Stock standard. 60 mg lithium carbonate + 60 ml water. Warm to 60 to 70°C. Add 100 mg uric acid powder. Dissolve. Add 2 ml formaline + 1 ml 50% acetic acid. Make the volume to 100 ml with water.
- *Working standard* Dilute 10 to 100 ml with water (10 mg/dl)

Procedure

Label three (12 × 100 mm) test tubes T (test) S (standard) and B (blank) and proceed as follows:

Pipette	T	S	B
Water (ml)	0.2	4.0	4.5
Serum (ml)	0.2	–	–
Standard (ml)	–	0.2	–
10% sodium tungstate (ml)	2.0 ml	0.25	0.25
2/3 N H_2SO_4 (ml)	0.25	0.25	0.25
Mix, stand for 10 minutes and centrifuge. To another set of 15 × 150 mm tubes, add			
Supernatant (ml)	3.0	3.0	3.0
Phosphotungstate reagent (ml)	1.0	1.0	1.0
Sodium carbonate (14%) ml	1.0	1.0	1.0

Mix after each addition. Stand at room temperature for 15 minutes. Read with in next 30 minutes at 710 nm or using red filter. Adjust the instruments at 0. OD with water.

Calculation

$$\text{Uric acid mg/dl} = \frac{\text{OD Test} - \text{OD Blank}}{\text{OD Std} - \text{OD Blank}} \times 5$$

Normal Values

Male : 2.5 to 7.0 mg/dl

Female : 1.5 to 6.0 mg/dl

Interpretation

- Increased values are seen in gout, leukemia, pneumonia and polycythemia.
- Low values may be seen in Wilson's disease and Fanconi's syndrome.

Other methods: Different modifications based on reaction of uric acid with phosphotungstic acid reagent are used.

Method utilizing the absorption at 293 nm before and after the action of enzyme uricase is also used.

Estimation of Serum Alkaline Phosphatase

It is an enzyme which catalyzes the breakdown of organic phosphate compounds. It has its optimum activity at an alkaline pH. It releases inorganic phosphate. Determination of alkaline phosphatase activity is useful in bone diseases and as liver function test.

Method (King and King)

Principle

Alkaline phosphate present in serum acts on the substrate disodium phenyl phosphate at pH 10. Phenol released during experimental period at 37°C is estimated and is measure of enzyme activity.

Reagents

- *Sodium carbonate/bicarbonate buffer*: Dissolve 6.36 gm of anhydrous sodium carbonate and 3.36 gm sodium bicarbonate in about 950 ml water. Adjust pH to 10.0 with 0.1N NaOH or HCl and dilute to 1 liter. Keep at 2 to 8°C.

- *Disodium phenyl phosphate (10 nM)*: 2.18 gm disodium phenyl phosphate is dissolved per liter. The solution is quickly brought to boil, cooled and store at 2 to 8°C in brown bottle (Add 4 ml/liter chloroform as preservative).
- *Sodium hydroxide (0.5N)*: 20 gm NaOH flakes or pellets weighed quickly and dissolved in about 900 ml water. The solution is cooled and volume made to 1 liter.
- *Sodium bicarbonate (0.5 N)*: 42 gm sodium bicarbonate/liter.
- *4-aminoantipyrine* 6 gm/liter in water (store in brown bottle).
- *Potassium ferricyanide*: 24 gm potassium ferricyanide/liter of water (store in brown bottle).
- *Stock phenol standard (100 mg/dl)*: 100 mg pure crystals of phenol dissolved per 100 ml 0.1N HCl (store at 2 to 8°C in brown bottle).
- *Working phenol standard (1 mg/dl)*: Dilute 1 to 100 ml with distilled water (store as earlier).

Procedure

Label 15 × 150 mm clean dry test tubes as T (test) C (control) S (standard) and B (blank) and proceed as follows. Mix thoroughly after each addition.

	T	C	S	B
Add buffer (ml)	1.0	1.0	1.1	1.1
Phenyl phosphate (ml)	1.0	1.0	–	–
Keep the (T) tube at 37°C for 3 minutes. Add 0.1 ml serum and incubate at 37°C for exact 15 minutes.				
Sodium hydroxide 0.5 N	0.8	0.8	0.8	0.8
Serum (ml)	–	0.1	–	–
Phenol working standard (ml)	–	–	1.0	–
Sodium bicarbonate (0.5 N) ml	1.2	1.2	1.2	1.2
4-Aminoantipyrine (ml)	1.0	1.0	1.0	1.0
Potassium ferricyanide (ml)	1.0	1.0	1.0	1.0

Take readings immediately at 510 to 520 nm or using green filter against water.

Calculation

Serum alkaline phosphatase activity (King Armstrong units/100 ml)

$$= \frac{\text{OD Test} - \text{OD Cont}}{\text{OD Std} - \text{OD Blank}} \times 10$$

(1 KA units is the production of 1 mg phenol in 15 minute at pH 10 and at 37°C).

Normal Values

Adults 3 to 13 KA units/dl
Children 7 to 27 KA units/dl
- Raised in Bone diseases (rickets, osteomalacia, bone tuberculosis, bone fracture, bone tumors, hyperparathyroid, obstructive jaundice due to gallstones, liver, carcinoma, carcinoma of head pancreas)
- Lowered in Paget's disease, malnutrition, scurvy, bone irradiation.
  Other methods measure the liberated in organic phosphate such as Bodansky's method.

Estimation of Serum Acid Phosphatase

Acid Phosphatase

It is an enzyme which catalyses the breakdown of organic phosphate compounds. Its optimum activity is at an acidic pH of 5-6. Determination of acid phosphatase activity is useful in diagnosis of cancer of prostate.

Method (King and Jegatheesan)

Principle

Same as in an alkaline phosphatase except that the reaction is carried at a pH of 5.0.

Reagents

- *Citrate buffer (pH 4.9)* Dissolve 42 gm of dry crystalline citric acid in about 500 ml water. Add 376 ml of 1 N NaOH. Adjust pH to 4.9-5 and dilute to 1 liter with water. Store at 2-8°C with few drops of chloroform as preservative.
- Other reagents are as in the estimation of alkaline phosphatase.

Procedure

The procedure of acid phosphatase estimation is similar to that of alkaline phosphatase except:

- Take 1.0 ml of citrate buffer in test and control and 1.2 ml in St and blank tubes in place of carbonate/bicarbonate buffer.
- Incubate at 37°C for exact 60 minutes and not for 15 minutes.

Calculations

Serum acid phosphatase activity (KA units/100 ml)

$$= \frac{\text{OD Test} - \text{OD Cont}}{\text{OD Std} - \text{OD Blank}} \times 5$$

(King Armstrong unit is defined as that activity which produces 1 mg of phenol in the test at 37°C in 1 hour).

To differentiate acid phosphatase of prostate origin from others, prepare a second T tube. Add 1 drop of tartrate solution (15% solution in water adjusted to pH 4.9 before adding serum. Follow the procedure exactly. Subtract the value of number 2 test from Number 1 test to get prostatic acid phosphatase value.

Normal Values

1.0 to 3.5 KA units mg/dl

Interpretation

Raised in prostatic carcinoma, after prostate massage, leukemia, Paget's disease, chronic liver diseases and breast cancer, etc.

Other methods measure the liberated inorganic phosphatase such as Bodansky method.

Estimation of Serum Amylase

Amylase is an enzyme found in pancreatic juice and saliva. A small quantity is found in serum. In pancreatitis and mump, larger quantities are found in blood and help in diagnosis of acute pancreatitis.

Somogyi Method

Principle

Serum is incubated with starch solution at a pH of 7.0. serum amylase hydrolyzes starch to maltase. The starch remaining unhydrolyzed is measured by blue color given by starch with iodine. Difference of blue color produced by original starch solution and after hydrolysis is a measure of enzyme activity.

Reagents

- Normal saline
- *Starch solution*: 100 mg/dl In 0.1% benzoic acid.
- *Buffer solution pH 7.0*: 1.736 gm anhydrous Na_2HPO_4 + 1.059 gm KH_2PO_4/liter, add 2 to 3 ml chloroform store at 2 to 8°C.
- *Buffered starch solution (prepared freshly)*: Mix 4 ml of 0.1% starch with 5.0 ml of buffer.
- *Iodine 0.1N*: Dissolve 24 gm potassium iodide in about 500 ml water add 12.7 gm iodine crystals and dissolve. Dilute to 1000 ml with water.
- *Iodine solution for use*: To 60 to 70 ml water, add 5 gm KI and dissolve. Add 10 ml of 0.1 N iodine. Mix and dilute to 100 ml with water.

Procedure

Add 0.1 ml serum to 0.9 ml of normal saline and mix. Label two 18 × 150 mm test tubes as test (T) or control (C) and proceed as follows:
1. Take 0.9 ml buffered starch in both T and C.
2. Warm T tube at 37°C for 2 to 3 minutes.
3. Add 0.1 ml diluted serum.
4. Incubate at 37°C for exact 15 minutes.
5. Cool quickly by immersing in ice cold water.
6. Add 8.6 ml water.
7. Add 0.4 ml 0.01 N iodine and mix.
8. Prepare the control similarly but adding diluted serum after step 7 above.

Compare the absorbance at 660 nm or using a red filter with water as blank.

Calculation

Serum amylase activity Somogyi units/100 ml =

$$= \frac{\text{OD of control} - \text{OD of test}}{\text{OD of control}} \times 800$$

A unit is defined as an activity which digests 1 mg of starch at pH 7.0 and 37°C in 1 hour.

Serum Glutamic Oxaloacetic Transaminase (SGOT) (Serum Aspartate Transaminase)

Aspartate transaminase is an enzyme widely distributed with high concentration in liver, heart, muscles, RBCs, etc. In the cells, the enzyme is required for the metabolism of amino acid aspartate. Normal serum has some basic levels of this enzyme but the concentration of enzyme increases after damage to the cardiac, liver and red blood cells and helps in the diagnosis of the myocardial infarction, hepatitis, etc.

Colorimetric DNPH Method

Principle

Aspartate transaminase present in serum acts in aspartate and transfers amino group to 2-oxoglutarate as follows:

$$\text{L-Aspartate} + \text{2-Oxoglutarate} \xrightarrow{\text{Asp. transaminase}} \text{L-Glutamate} + \text{Oxaloacetate}$$

Oxaloacetate formed reacts with 2, 4-dinitrophenyl hydrazine to form a complex which is in alkaline medium is converted to brown color. The concentration of the color is measured at 505 nm.

Reagents

- *Phosphate buffer pH 7.4*: Dissolve 5.95 gm Na_2HPO_4 anhydrous (8.82 gm $Na_2HPO_2 \cdot 2H_2O$) + 1.1 gm NaH_2PO_4 in about 480 ml water. Adjust pH to 7.4 with either salt added in small amounts. Dilute to 500 ml, store at 2 to 8°C.
- *Buffered substrate*: Dissolve 29.2 mg of 2-oxoglutarate and 2.66 gm of DL aspartic acid in about 20 ml 1-LN NaOH. Adjust to pH 7.4 with more 1 N NaOH. Transfer to a 100 ml volumetric flask. Dilute to 100 ml with phosphate buffer. Add 1 ml chloroform. Store at 2 to 8°C.
- *Sodium hydroxide 1N*: 4 gm NaOH/100 ml.
- *Sodium hydroxide 0.4N*: 16 gm NaOH/L.
- *Color reagent*: 2, 4-dinitrophenyl hydrazine. Dissolve 20 mg DNPH in 100 ml 1 N HCl Store at 2 to 8°C.
- *Pyruvate standard solution*: 2 mmol/liter. Dissolve 22 mg sodium pyruvate in 100 ml phosphate buffer. Keep frozen in small volumes.

Procedure

Label three test tubes T (test) C (control) and B (blank) and proceed as follows:

Section 7: Biochemistry

	T	C	B
Add buffered substrate (ml)	0.5	0.5	0.5
Incubate at 37°C for 5 minutes			
Patient serum (ml)	0.1	–	–
Water (ml)	–	–	0.1
Incubate at 37°C for 60 minutes			
DNPH (ml)	0.5	0.5	0.5
Patient serum	–	0.1	–
Keep at room temperature for 20 minutes			
0.4 N NaOH (ml)	5.0	5.0	5.0

Take readings after 5 minutes with green filter or using 505 nm wavelength. Set zero with reagent blank.

Use a calibration curve to calculate the values.

Take five clean test tubes. label them a 1, 2, 3, 4 and 5. Pipette into each in the following order:

Tube No		1	2	3	4	5
Equivalent of enzyme activity/(ml) (SGOT)	SGOT	0	24	61	114	190
	SGPT	0	28	57	97	150
Buffered substrate (ml)		0.5	0.45	0.4	0.35	0.3
Pyruvate standard (ml)		–	0.05	0.1	0.15	0.2
Distilled water (ml)		0.1	0.1	0.1	0.1	0.1
DNPH (color reagent) (ml)		0.5	0.5	0.5	0.5	0.5
Mix well and allow to stand at room temperature for 20 minutes.						
Sodium hydroxide 0.4 N (ml)		5.0	5.0	5.0	5.0	5.0

Mix well and take readings after 5 minutes at 505 nm or using green filter.

Plot a graph, with the enzyme activity on X-axis and corresponding OD of tubes 2 to 5 on Y-axis, adjusting O with tube number 1. Find out the value of sample from graph using ODT-OD control as the OD of test.

Normal Values

8 to 40 U/ml

Interpretations

Raised values are seen in myocardial infarction various types of liver diseases, muscular dystrophies and hemolysis.

Serum Glutamic Pyruvate Transaminase (SGPT) (Serum Alanine Transaminase)

Alanine transaminase is also widely distributed. Its activity is higher in liver than that of AST. Normal function of ALT in cells is in the metabolism of amino acid alanine. The enzyme leaks into blood on damage to the cell. Estimation of the serum enzyme is particularly beneficial in acute hepatitis.

Colorimetric 2, 4-Dinitrophenyl Hydrazine (DNPH) Method

Principle

Alanine transaminase present in serum on incubation with its substrate alanine transfers the amino group from alanine to oxoglutarate. Alanine is converted to pyruvate which combines with DNPH to form a complex, which gives a brown color in alkaline medium. The concentration of color is measured at 505 nm and is a measure of enzyme activity.

Reagents

- *Phosphate buffer*: As in SGOT estimation.
- *Buffered substrate*: Dissolve 1.88 gm of DL, alanine instead of DL, aspartate, and proceed as in serum glutamate oxaloacetate transaminase (SGOT) estimation. Other reagents are similar to SGOT estimation.

Procedure

Follow the procedure of SGOT estimation except:
- Use buffered substrate the alanine.
- Incubate at 37°C for 30 minutes instead of 60 minutes.

Calibration curve: Prepare calibration curve as in SGOT. Use buffered substrate of ALT. Plot a graph as per the readings against SGPT units.

Note: In case of high ALT or AST activity in sample, use suitably diluted serum with normal saline, and repeat the assay. Multiply the results with the dilution factor.

Normal Values
5 to 35 U/ml.

Interpretation
Increased values are found in liver disease, myocardial infarction, muscular dystrophy, etc.

Other methods: Continuous monitoring method or kinetic methods using the absorption of light at 340 nm by reduced NAD (NADH), and not by NAD.

SGPT (Alanine Transaminase)

$$\text{L-alanine} + \text{2-oxoglutarate} \xrightarrow{\text{SGPT}} \text{Pyruvate} + \text{L-glutamate}$$

$$\text{Pyruvate} + \text{NADH} + \text{H}^+ \xrightarrow{\text{Lactate dehydrogenase}} \text{L-Lactate} + \text{NAD}^+$$

SGOT (Aspartate Transaminase)

$$\text{L-asparate} + \text{2-oxoglutarate} \xrightarrow{\text{SGOT}} \text{Oxaloacetate} + \text{L-glutamate}$$

$$\text{Oxaloacetate} + \text{NADH} + \text{H}^+ \xrightarrow{\text{Malate dehydrogenase}} \text{Malate} + \text{NHD}^+$$

The reduction in absorption is continuously measured at 340 nm in a spectrophotometer and is a measure of SGOT or SGPT activity.

Automation in Clinical Laboratory

Introduction
Automation is the mechanization of the steps in a procedure. It not only saves labor but also allows reliable quality control measures to be imposed strongly. The automation in clinical laboratory has advantages including the increased accuracy, less discrepancy in results, better quality control, reduced subjective errors and the use of smaller quantities of samples and reagents.

Classification of Automation
The automated system is grouped into following types:

Continuous Flow Analysis (Figs. 8.2 and 8.3)

This is the first automated system introduced by Technicon (USA) in 1960s which has since been followed by other systems. In this system, liquid specimen, reagents and diluents are pumped through a system of continuous flow tubing. Samples are introduced in a sequential manner, following each other through the same network. A series of air bubbles separate and clean the media. The commonly used models are SMA 6/60 and 12/60, which process 60 specimens per hoyr and report the results of 6 and 12 parameters simultaneously. This system is ideal for larger laboratories.

Disadvantages
- The physician may not be interested in all the tests reported by the instrument.

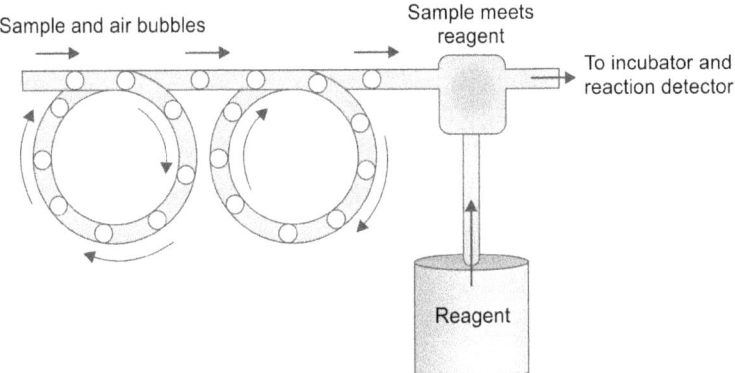

Fig. 8.2: Continuous flow analyzer

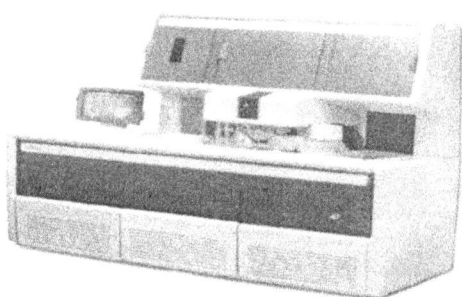

Fig. 8.3: Continuous flow analyzer

- The instrument does not report the test, which the physician may be interested in.

Discrete Analysis (Fig. 8.4)

In this system, each sample is separated along with the accompanying reagent. This can be used both for special tests and routine tests. It is ideal for smaller laboratories. The commonly used models for this system are Clinicon (Boehringer Mannheim) and Auto Pacer (Miles of India Ltd)

Centrifugal Analyzer (Fig. 8.5)

This is the recent automated system used. In this system, the specimens and the corresponding reagents are placed in their places on the special

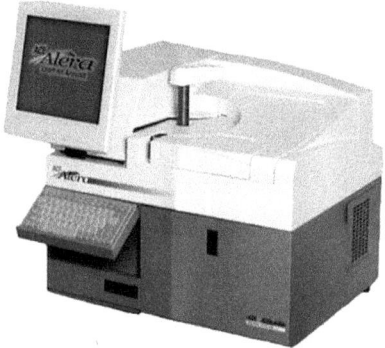

Fig. 8.4: Discrete analyzer

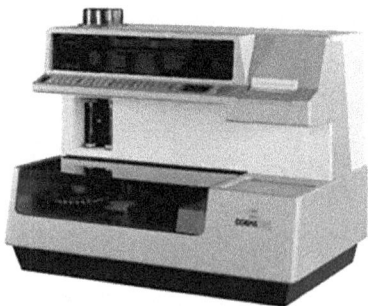

Fig. 8.5: Centrifugal analyzer

centrifuge head, the machine is run and the force generated by the centrifugation transfers the reagents and the specimen to a cuvette for chemical reaction to occur. The optical measurements are made while the cuvette is in motion (2500 rpm). It is the most useful in performing enzyme assays.

Random Access Analyzer

Random access analyzers perform analyzes on a batch of specimens sequentially with each specimen analyzed for a different selection of tests. The tests performed in the random access analyzers are selectable through the use of different containers of liquid reagents, different reagent packs, or different reagent tablets depending upon the analyzer. This approach permits measurement of a variable number and variety of analytes in each specimen. Profiles or group of tests are defined for a specimen at the time the requested tests are entered into analyzer by means of a keyboard, by instruction from a laboratory information system in conjunction with barcoding on the specimen tube or by operator selection of appropriate reagent packs. Like centrifugal analyzers, random access analyzers incorporate computers and are able to take multiple absorbance or reflectance measurements for each assay.

Steps of Automation in Biochemical Analysis

The steps are divided as below:
- Sample handling
- Sample processing
- Reagent handling
- Analytical procedure
- Reaction analysis or sensing
- Calculation
- **Sample handling and sample processing:** The specimens are manually labeled, centrifuged and divided into aliquots if tests for more than one work station have been requested. This manual processing also removes the specimens which are not acceptable for the analysis (e.g. hemolyzed or lipemic specimens, presence of debris) and reviews the request form received with the specimen. Extreme care is needed in this step to avoid mislabeling of patient samples or their aliquots.

Section 7: Biochemistry

In automated systems, the sample holding containers must be placed in the same order and the laboratory professional must note down the order of the arrangement clearly. Some laboratories prefer to number the sample cups so that if they are misplaced, they can be put into the proper slot. In most automated system, the samples are held in small cups which are placed on a circular tray. The slots are sequentially numbered. An automatic pipette can be used for taking aliquots of specimens into the sample cups. Fresh tip is used for each sample. In continuous flow analysis, the requisite amount of specimen is picked up by the sampler while in others an aliquot of the specimen may have to be manually placed. Probes used in the automated systems for picking up specimen must be thoroughly washed, preferably with a diluent, before the following specimen is drawn. The convenient way is to dispense the specimen and then the diluent to avoid the carry over effect.

Protein causes major interference in many analyses. In the continuous flow analysis system, dialyzer removes the protein from the specimen. However, the dialyzer is not used for protein determination. In other automated system, there is no such step that removes protein from the sample. The other systems use a method that will be least interfered by the presence of protein or they use a more sensitive method or they add appropriate chemicals to remove the protein. Some discrete analyzers read the absorbances with two wavelengths that helps to reduce the effects of protein.

- **Reagent handling:** Most chemical reactions require the combining of reagent and sample in exact amounts. This is called proportioning. In continuous flow analysis, the diameter of the tube regulates the volume of the reagent fluid picked up, the amount of specimen. The dwelling time of the probe inside the specimen container determines the amount of specimen picked up. The rate of flow for all fluids is the same. A single peristaltic pump is used for drawing the fluids. For the discrete system, a single probe may measure the volumes of specimens and reagents but the dwelling time in them varies. Individual automatic dispensers are also used in some discrete systems where syringes and volumetric overflow devices are used to dispense requisite quantities of sample and reagent into test tubes or containers.

Reagents can be dispensed directly from bulk containers supplied by the manufacturer or reconstituted in the laboratory. Those manufacturers who are able to supply dry reagents or provide

the necessary formula for the preparation of reagents within the laboratory, will be the most successful in marketing their goods in the developing countries.
- **Analytical procedure:** Mixing of reagents with the specimen is a vital component of biochemical analysis. In continuous flow system, it is done through glass coils where the liquid rotates and both specimen and reagents fall through one another during their rise and fall through the loop. In the discrete systems, other methods are adopted-vibration, slewing action, centrifugal rotation (in centrifugal analyzers), vortexing, pressing and releasing of plastic bags which receive the fluids and ultrasonic waves.

  Automated incubation is merely a delay station where the test mixture is allowed to react. The chamber where the incubation is held is heated to the desired temperature by the use of heating block, air, water bath or oil bath. To sustain the advantage of speedy multiple analyses, the reaction is not taken to completion. Rather, the rate of the reaction can be measured and the values after the completion of the reaction are extrapolated. The instruments may also delay the measurement for a pre-determined length of time or present the reaction mixtures for measurement at constant intervals of time. In continuous flow analysis, all measurements are made against a standard and as the procedures are precisely timed, the result of the standard is highly reproducible even if the measurement is made much before the completion of the reaction. In the discrete system, there are a number of delay stations before the readings are taken.
- **Reaction analysis or sensing:** After the reaction is completed, there must be a sensing device (colorimeter) to measure the change such as development of color. The sensing can be done in the original site where the reaction occurred (internal) or taken into another vessel (external) to make the measurements. In the continuous flow analysis, the reagent stream under analysis flow continuously through the flow cell which acts like a cuvette. The air bubbles are removed by the debubbler before the reacted solution enters the flow cell for photometric measurements. The sensing device converts the optical response into electrical impulses which are then sent to the read out device. The read out device can be the strip chart on which the results are traced or on the digital display.

  Chemical reactions can be monitored either at one time point or at many. Commonly, single point monitoring is used for end point (or mid point) analysis in which the reaction has gone to completion

or the instrument extrapolates the value. Multiple point monitoring is done in case of kinetic studies (enzyme activity).
- **Calculation of results:** In the automated system, the results are automatically computed from the response of the sensor and finally printed out in appropriate units. The printing can be done directly on patient's request slip (or reporting slip) or on the laboratory form. In order to avoid transcription errors, it is advisable that multiple copies of the print out should be made so that different copies of the same report can be routed to different destination-financial office, physician, patient's record, laboratory record and others.

Quality Control in Automated System

Automated systems are not free from errors. In fact, they frequently render a false sense of security among the users and the results may be far from reliable. The system must be frequently subjected to quality control procedures using control sera. Control runs should be done in the beginning of each day and the result is plotted on the quality control chart.

Advantages of Automation
- Increase the number of tests by one person in a given period of time
- Minimize the variations in results from one person to another
- Minimize errors found in manual analyses—equipment variations —pipettes
- Use *less* sample and reagent for each test

Disadvantages of Automation
- Vary with the instrument type
- High initial cost: Generally cost of equipment, maintenance, amount of QC (Quality Control)
- Also technologist must be kept knowledgeable and careful in setup and operations
- Decreases work opportunities of man power.

Appendices

APPENDIX 1

Hematological Values

Sl. No.	Normal values	Increased	Decreased
1.	Hemoglobin (gm/l00 ml) Men = 13.5 to 18 Women = 11.5 to 16.4 Infant = 13 to 19 Children (10 years) = 12	Dehydration Polycythemia	Anemia
2	Red blood cell Total count per cub mm Men = 4.5 to 6.5 Women = 3.9 to 5.6 Infant = 4 to 6 (cord blood) Children = (10 years) 4.2	Polycythemia Dehydration Anorexia CCF CHD High altitude	Anemia
3.	Reticulocyte % RBC Adult = 0 to 2.2 Infant (cord blood) = 2.6	Pernicious anemia Treatment of anemia Hemolytic anemia After acute hemorrhage	
4.	Packed cell volume (PCV)% Men = 4 to 54 Women = 36 to 47 Infant = 44 to 62 Children (10 years) = 37.5	Dehydration without anemia Infancy Polycythemia Addison disease	Anemia
5.	Mean cell volume (MCV) cubic micron Adult= 70 to 96	Pernicious anemia Liver disease Sprue Tropical macrocyte Anemia	Iron deficiency anemia Acholuric jaundice Polycythemia vera

6.	Mean cell hemoglobin (MCH) µg Adult = 27 to 32		
7.	Mean cell Hemoglobin concentration (%) Adult= 32 to 35	Normal in aplastic anemia and pernicious anemia	Iron deficiency anemia Acholuric jaundice??
8.	Total white cell count (per cubic mm) Adults = 5000 to 10,000 Children = 5000 to 14000	Pyogenic infection Infectious mononucleosis Whooping cough Leukemoid reaction Infarction hemolysis	Typhoid fever Virus infection Kala-azar Chronic malaria Agranulocytosis Anaphylactic shock hypersplenism
9.	Platelets (per cubic mm) 1,50,000 to 4,00,000	After delivery Hemorrhage Thrombocytopenia After splenectomy After exercise	Pancytopenia Hypersplenism Purpura?? Pernicious anemia Acute leukemia
10.	Erythrocyte sedimentation rate (Westergren method) mm in one hour Men = 3 to 5 mm Women = 4 to 7 mm	Febrile condition Tuberculosis Rheumatism Thrombosis?? Leukemia Thrombocytopenia Hemorrhagic status DIC Prothrombin deficiency	

Biochemical Values

	Normal values	Increased	Decreased
Blood glucose (fasting)	80 to 120 mg%	Diabetic mellitus Certain cerebral lesion Hyperpituitarism	Sprue Hyperinsulinism
Urea	15 to 30 mg%	Primary renal disease Dehydration Intestinal obstruction Urinary tract infection	Low protein diet Severe liver damage
Urea nitrogen	10 to 15 mg%	As in urea	As in urea
Nonprotein nitrogen	20 to 40 mg%	As in urea except liver disease	As in urea
Uric acid	2 to 5 mg%	Gout Chronic leukemia Polycythemia Lead poisoning	As in urea
Creatine	1 to 2 mg	Oliguria Renal failure Anemia Urinary tract obstruction	Loss of gastrointestinal secretion Uremic acidosis Addison's disease
Creatinine	0.7 to 2 mg%		
Chloride	0.5 to 110 mg%		
Potassium (serum)	3.5 to 5.5 MEq/L	Addison disease Cushing syndrome Renal failure	Chronic diarrhoea Recovery phase of diabetic ketoacidosis
Sodium (serum)	137 to 147 mEq/L	Acute nephritis Cardiac failure	Addison crisis excessive loss of body fluid
Calcium (serum)	7 to 11 mg% (4.5 to 5.7 mEq/L)	Hyperparathyroidism Hypervitaminosis D Multiple myelomatosis Hyperproteinemia	Hypoparathyroidism Hypoproteinemia Uremia Rickets Osteomalacia

Test	Normal range	Increased in	Decreased in
Acid phosphatase	0.5 to 3.25 KA unit 0 to Bodansky units	Prostate cancer with metastasis (100 units and above) Hyperparathyroidism Paget disease	
Alkaline phosphatase	3 to 15 KA unit/dl	Liver diseases Hyperparathyroidism Obstructive jaundice Secondary carcinomatosis of bone osteomalacia	
Total protein (plasma)	6 to 18 gm%	Multiple myelomatosis Diabetic coma	Starvation Malnutrition Chronic liver disease Chronic kidney disease
Albumin	3.5 to 5.8 gm%	Anhydremia	Malnutrition Chronic liver disease Subacute and chronic kidney disease
Globulin	2 to 2.5 gm%	Chronic liver disease Kala-azar Tuberculosis Sarcoidosis Multiple myelomatosis Chronic malaria Kidney disease with albuminemia	
Bilirubin	0.1 to 0.8 mg%	Jaundice	
Cholesterol (serum)	150 to 250 mg/dl	Obstructive jaundice Nephrosis Diabetic mellitus Hypothyroidism	Hyperthyroidism Chronic anemia
Amylase (serum)	60 to 100 mg/100 ml	Acute hemorrhagic pancreatitis Pancreatic calculi with pancreatitis	
Serum iron	60 to 100 mg/100 ml		Iron deficiency anemia

CSF			
Protein	25 to 45 mg/100 ml	Meningitis Poliomyelitis Froin's syndrome	
Calcium	0.1 to 0.7 g/24 hr	Cushing syndrome Hyperadrenalism	Addison disease Simmonds' disease
Chloride	10 to 15 g/24 hr		
Nitrogen	12 to 18 g/24 hr		
Urea	20 to 35 g/24 hr		
Urobilinogen	0.4 mg/100 ml		

APPENDIX 2

Electron Microscope

Highlights
- Uses a beam of accelerated electrons as a source of illumination
- First invented by Ernst Ruska in 1931
- Two types
    1. Transmission electron microscope (TEM)
    2. Scanning electron microscope (SEM)

Transmission Electron Microscope (TEM)

It is a technique in which a beam of electrons are transmitted through an ultra thin specimen.

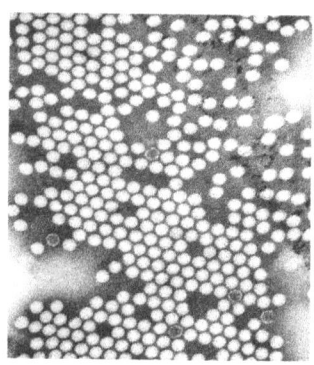
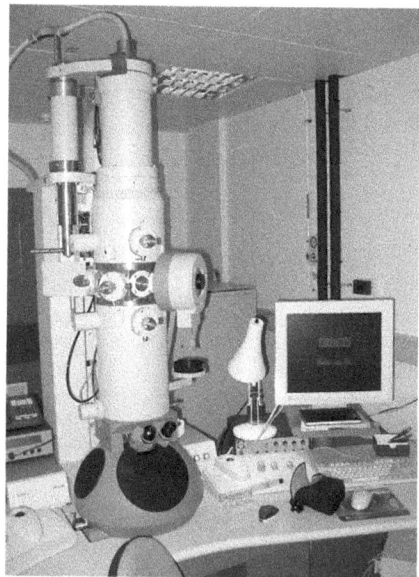

Parts of TEM
- Electron gun
- Electromagnetic lenses
- Specimen holder
- Image viewing and recording system

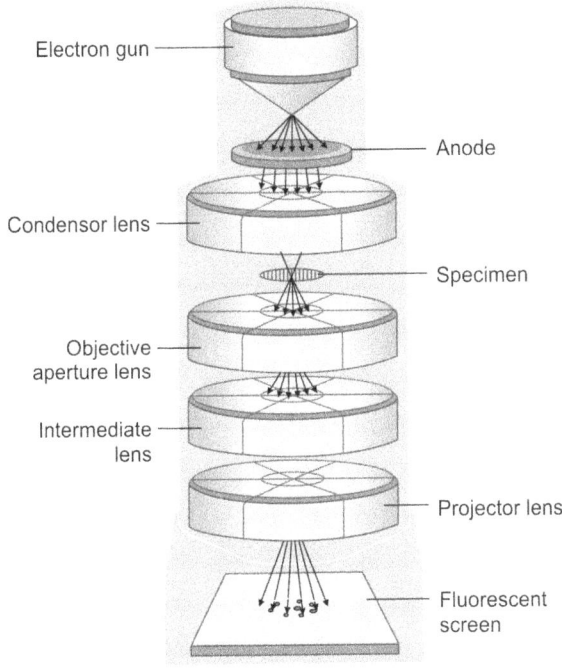

Working Principle of TEM

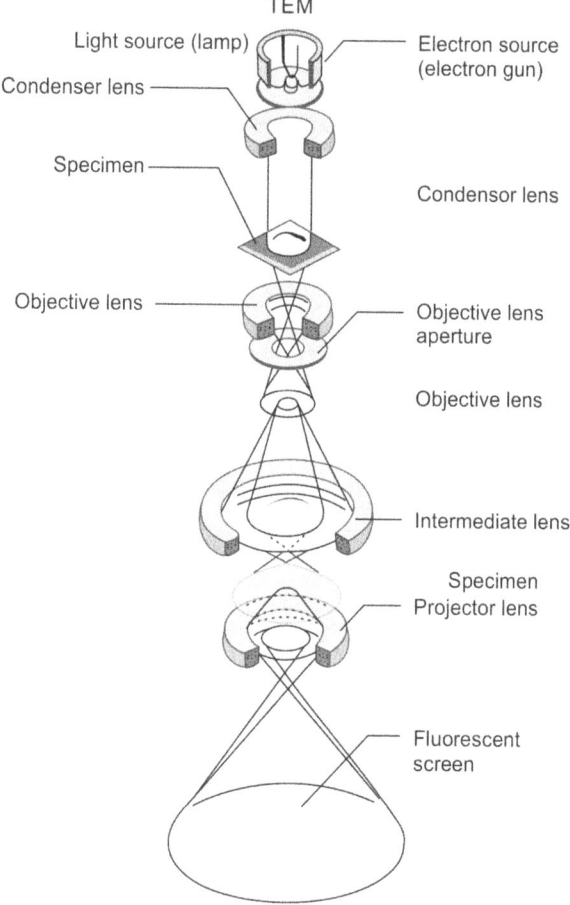

Appendices

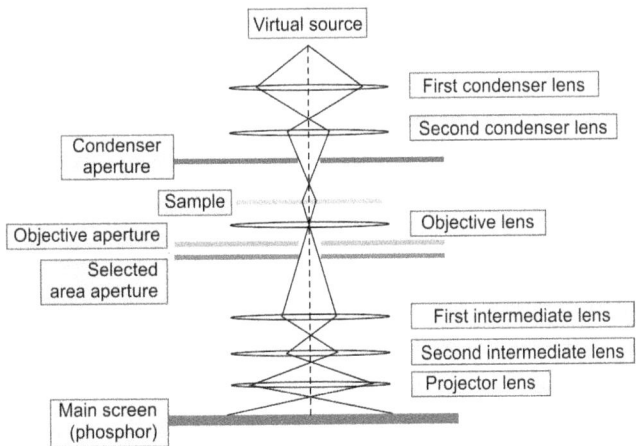

Sample Preparation

- Cleaning the surface of the specimen
- Primary fixation of the specimen
- Rinsing of the specimen
- Secondary fixation of the specimen
- Dehydration
- Infiltration of specimen with transitional solvent
- Sectioning and staining of the specimen

Applications

- Used as diagnostic tool
- Cellular tomography
- Studies of tumor cell ultrastructure
- To study impacts of environmental pollution on different levels of biological organization

Advantages

- Offer very powerful magnification and resolution
- Utilized in variety of different scientific, educational and industrial fields
- Provide information on element and compound structure

Disadvantages

- Difficult to produce thin sample

- Time consuming process
- Structure of sample may be change during preparation process.

Scanning Electron Microscope (SEM)

- EM that produces image of a sample by scanning it with a focused beam of electrons
- Electrons interact with atoms in sample, producing various signals that contain information about sample's surface topography and composition

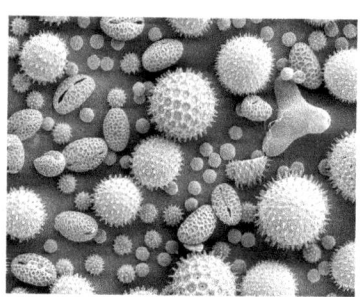

Parts of SEM
- Electron gun
- Electron lenses
  - Condenser lens
  - Objective lens

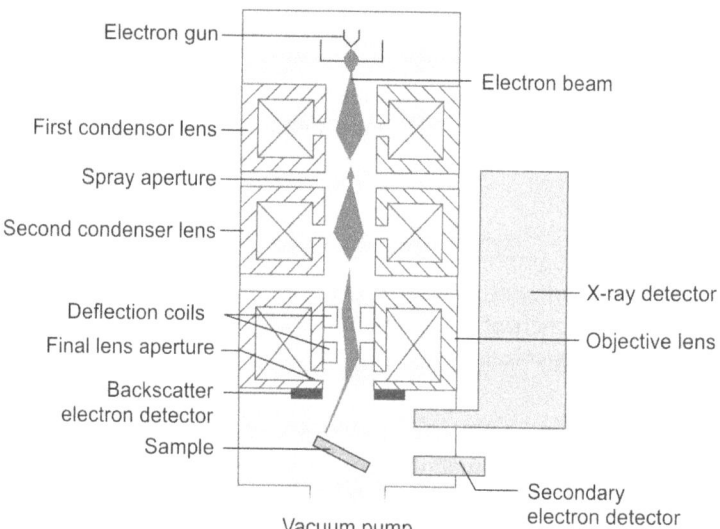

Working of SEM

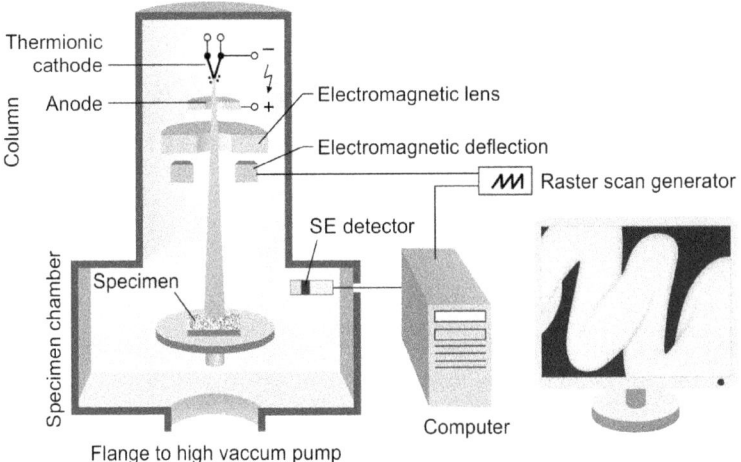

Sample Preparation
- Fixation and dehydration
- Drying with hexamethyldisilazane (HMDS) and t-Butanol
- Coating with gold/Palladium using sputter coater
- Image processing

APPENDIX 3

Protocol for Conducting COVID-19 PCR

Sample Aliquot Preparation Protocol for COVID-19 Nitrile Gloves

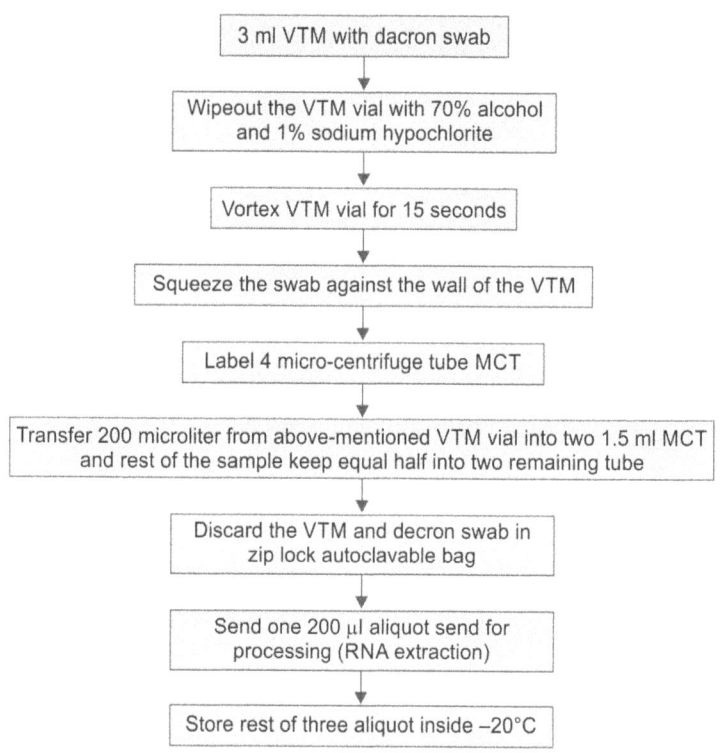

Reagent Preparation of High Pure NA Kit

- **Proteinase K:** Dissolve Pk/carrier RNA to proteinase dissolve buffer
- **Buffer VLE:** Add 18 ml of isopropanol
- **Buffer CE:** Add 60 ml of isopropanol
- **Buffer AVE:** Ready to use
- **Storage:** Proteinase k 20°C and remaining room temperature

Sample Preparation

If immediate process sample may collected in 500 µl of NS, for preservation purpose VTM should be used.

Preparation of Master Mix

- **Personnel:** Microbiologist
- **PPE:** Disposable gown, N95 mask, hair net, face shield, gloves, and shoe cover.
- The master mix checklist should be verified.
- Proceed according to the provided master mix protocol.

Master Mix Protocol

Reagents	Volume/µl
PCR reaction liquid A	17
PCR reaction liquid B	2
PCR reaction liquid C	1
Total	20

Template Addition

- **Personnel:** Microbiologist
- **PPE:** Disposable gown, N95 mask, hair net, face shield, gloves, and shoe cover.
- Proceed according to the provided protocol.

Template Addition Protocol

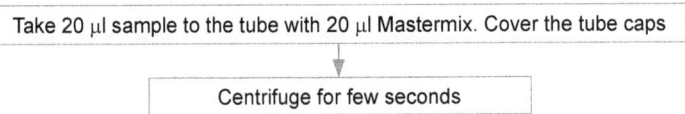

PCR Run

- **Personnel:** Microbiologist
- **PPE:** Disposable gown, disposable surgical mask, hair net, face shield, gloves, and shoe cover.
- Proceed according to the provided RT-PCR protocol.

RT-PCR Protocol

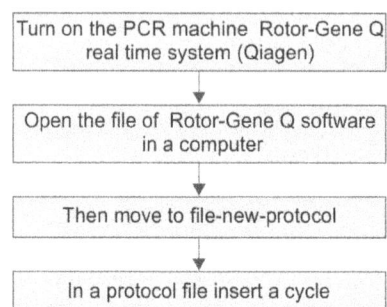

Step	Temperature	Time	Cycles
RT incubation	50°C	30 min	1
Enzyme activation	95°C	3 min	1
Denaturation	95°C	5 sec	40
Annealing and extension	55°C	30 sec	

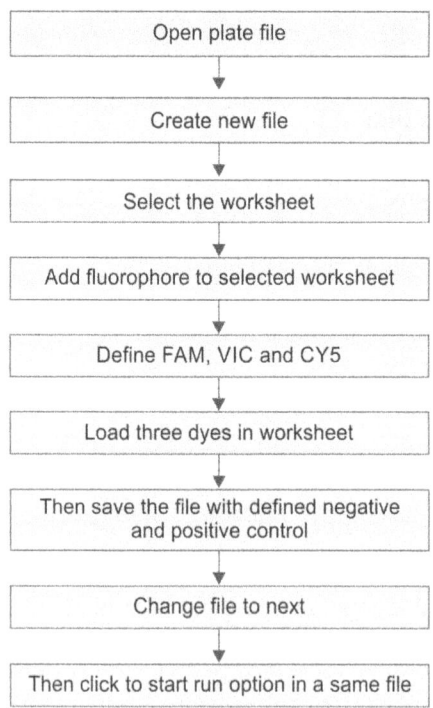

Components	Per RXN μl	Cycling condition	
Combined primer probe		Hold 1: 50°C for 30 minutes	Positive
Mix in well		Hold 2: 95°C for 3 minutes	FAM: ≤38 JOE: ≤38
		Cycle –45 95°C for 5 sec	Cy5: Not required
		55°C for 32 sec	Negative FAM: >38
		Reporter dye : FAM : VIC : Cy5	VIC: >38 Cy5: ≤33
		(quencher dye none)	Re test : FAM : VIC
			Re test : FAM : VIC : Cy5

APPENDIX 4

Bactec

- Based on fluorescent technology in detecting growth of microbes.
- Each vials contains a chemical sensor, i.e. liquid emulsion sensor.

Composition of Bactec Blood Culture Vials

The composition of BACTEC plus aerobic/F culture vials is as follows:

List of ingredients	BD BACTEC plus aerobic/F
Processed water	30 mL w/v
Soyabean-Casein digest broth	3.0%
Yeast extract	0.25%
Amino acids	20%
Sugar	0.2%
Vitamins	0.025%
Sodium polyanethol sulfonate (SPS)	0.05%
Antioxidants reductants	0.005%
Nonionic adsorbing resin	13.4%
Cation exchange resin	0.9%

Working Principle

- Growing organisms metabolize nutrients, releasing CO_2 into the medium.
- A dye in sensor at bottom of culture bottles will react with CO_2.
- This modulates the amount of light that is absorbed by a fluorescent material in sensor.
- Photodetectors measure the level of fluorescence, which corresponds to the amount of CO_2 released by the organisms.

Appendices

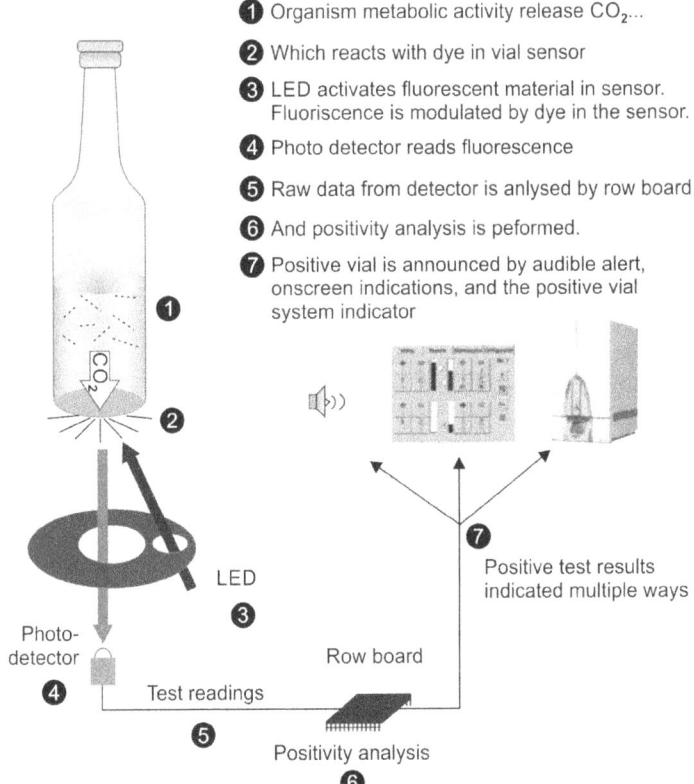

1. Organism metabolic activity release CO_2...
2. Which reacts with dye in vial sensor
3. LED activates fluorescent material in sensor. Fluoriscence is modulated by dye in the sensor.
4. Photo detector reads fluorescence
5. Raw data from detector is anlysed by row board...
6. And positivity analysis is peformed.
7. Positive vial is announced by audible alert, onscreen indications, and the positive vial system indicator

Positive test results indicated multiple ways

LED
Photo-detector
Test readings
Row board
Positivity analysis

Name of the medium	Use
BD BACTEC™ plus aerobic medium	All-purpose medium capable of supporting the growth of aerobic and facultative organisms
BD BACTEC™ plus anaerobic medium	All-purpose medium for common obligate anaerobic and facultative organisms
BD BACTEC™ peds plus media	Accommodate small volume and optimally direct common pediartic and on-pediatric organisms
BD BACTEC™ lytic anaerobic media	Increase the detection and recovery of anaerobes contains detergent to lyse RBC's and WBC's
BD BACTEC™ standard aerobic media	Recovery of bacteria and yeast from the blood
BD BACTEC™ standard anaerobic media	Recovery of anaerobic organisms from the blood

Advantages

- Continuous monitoring instrument
- Provides advance algorithms for each media types, for special circumstances such as low blood volume, pediatric specimens or to detect slow growing organisms
- Provide rapid detection of pathogens
- Decrease laboratory work

Disadvantages

- Expensive
- Limited selection of medium
- Inability to observe colony morphology

VITEK 2 Compact System

- An automated system used for bacterial identification and antimicrobial susceptibility testing
- Uses advanced colorimetry technology to determine individual biochemical reactions contained in a variety of microbe identification cards
- It uses colorimetric reagent card containing 64 wells
- Substrates in the well measure various metabolic activities such as acidification, alkalinization, enzyme hydrolysis
- Reaction pattern obtained from test organisms is compared with database
- It works on the principle of microbroth dilution
- The wells in the card contain doubling dilution of antimicrobial agents

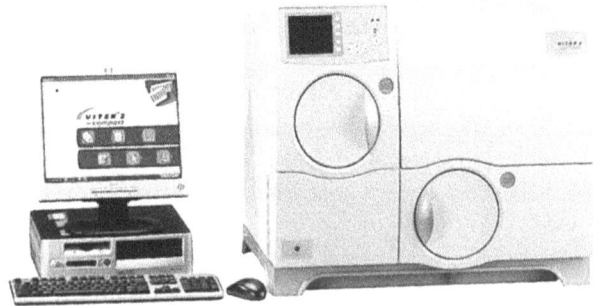

Components

- VITEK 2 compact
- Compact workstation
- Barcode scanner
- Test cassettes
- DensiCHEK plus

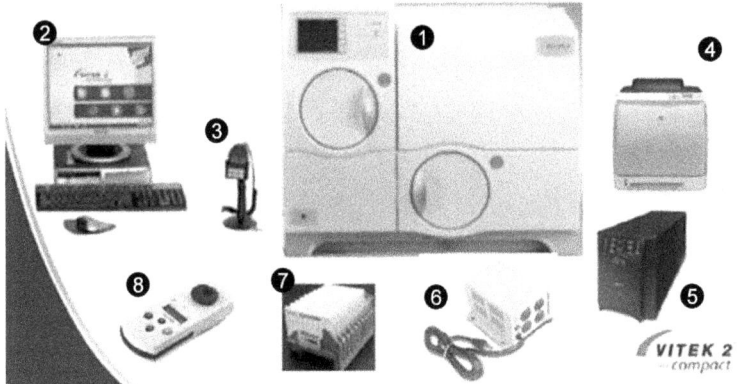

- Currently 4 reagent cards available
  1. GP—gram-negative fermenting and non-fermenting bacilli
  2. GP—gram-positive cocci and non-spore-forming bacilli
  3. YST—yeast and yeast-like organisms
  4. BCL—garm-positive spore-forming bacilli

Advantages

- Significant reduction in handling time
- Easy to handle
- Rapid and accurate identification

Index

Page numbers followed by *f* refer to figure.

A

ABO blood grouping
   indirect grouping 188
   method of 187
   slide method 187
   system 186
   tube technique 187
Abscess 100
Absolute eosinophil count 171
   procedure 172
Absolute methanol 229
Absorbance 144
Acetic acid 15
Acid
   citrate dextrose 177
   ethanol 15
   phosphatase 234
      procedure of 234
   reagent stock 220
Acidosis 74
Agglutination reactions 135
Airways tube 109
Alanine transaminase 240
Albert staining 107, 108
   principle 107
   procedure 108
Albumin 74, 147, 225
   BCG method 225
   in blood 224
Alkaline
   phosphatase 232
   phosphate 232
   picrate method 222
Alpha-hemolysis 122
Ammonium 177
Ampoules 110
Amyloid, stain for 210
Amyloidosis 225
Analytic balance 51*f*
   construction of 51
Analytical unit 54*f*
Analyzer operational systems 55
Ancylostoma duodenale 132

Anticoagulants 177
Antistreptolysin-O 139
   principle 139
   procedure 139
   requirements 139
   test 136
Arterial blood 176
Ascaris lumbricoides 133
Aspartate transaminase 240
Aspirated material, staining of 205
Autoanalyzer 53, 54*f*
   advantages 55
   analytical unit 53
   characteristics 55
   control unit 53
   disadvantages 56
   precautions 56
   procedure 55
Autoclave 42
   construction 42
   operation of 43
Automated system, quality control in 246
Automatic tissue processing unit 198*f*
Automation 240
   advantages of 246
   classification of 240
   disadvantages of 246

B

Bacilli 102, 103*f*
   shapes of 104*f*
Bactec 262
   blood culture vials, composition of 262
Bacteria 99
   culturing of 112
   demonstration of 104, 105
   description of 121
   examination of 102
   morphology of 102
   produce disease 100
   transmission of 99
Bacterial food, requirements for 112
Bacterial growth 117*f*, 118*f*

Bacterial infections 59
Bacteriological examination of drinking water, procedure for 126
Bacteriology 99
   laboratory 100
Balance 50
   analytic 50
   care of 52
   rough 50
   working of 52
Barium chloride aqueous solution 16
Basophil 169f
   cells 170
Bedding 110
Bedpans 110
Benedict qualitative solution 16
Benzidine test 87
Benzoic acid 216
Bicarbonate buffer 232
Bile
   pigments 75
      detection of 75
   salts 75
   solubility test 122
Bilirubin standard 229
Biochemical analysis, automation in 243
Biochemical test 118, 121, 122
Biochemical values 249
Biochemistry 215
Biological safety cabinet 43, 47
Biuret blank 224
Biuret reagent 224
Bladder cells 77
Bleeding time 175
   procedure 175
Blood
   A group 186
   AB group 186
   agar 115
   B group 186
   cast 79, 80f
   cholesterol estimation 227
   collection of 175, 189
   creatinine estimation 222
   cross-matching of 190
   functions of 147
   grouping 186
   O group 186
   pipette 159f
   preservation of 185
   smear, Leishman's staining of 169f
   spill 110
   stained linen 111
   sugar level 217
   urea estimation 220
Blood bank 185
   designing 185
   location 185
   organization of 185
Blood donors
   cell suspension 191
   selection of 189
Blood glucose
   estimation of 215
   levels, methods for estimation of 217
Blood transfusion 183, 186
   reactions, types of 191
Bodansky's method 234
Body fluids 69
Bone marrow
   aspiration
      procedure 181
      sites of 180
   biopsy 182
   examination 180
   hemosiderin in 182
   smear, examination of 181
Borax, standardization against 27
Borrelia 103
Breast cancer 235
Buffered starch solution 236
Buffered substrate 239
Burns 225

C

Calcium
   hydrogen phosphate 81f
   oxalate 79, 81f
Cancer cells 83
Capillary blood 176
   technique 176
Capillary method 173
Caraway methods 230
Carbol fuchsin 16, 17
Carotid body tumor 203
Cary-Blair transport medium 17
Catalase test 118, 121
Catheter 111
Cell 95
   composition 182
Cellular structure 182
Centrifugal analyzer 242, 242f, 245
Centrifuge machine 48, 49f
   construction 49
   precautions 50

Index

types of 50
use of 49
Cerebrospinal fluid 81, 100
   chemical examination 83, 85
   collection of specimen 82
   cytological examination 82, 85
   examination of 81
     reporting of 85
   features of 82
   functions of 81
   microbiological examination 86
   physical examination 82, 85
   staining 85
Cheatle forceps 111
Chloride estimation 84
Chocolate agar 115
Cholera 99
   bacilli 124
Cholesterol 227
   esters 228
Christensen's urease medium test 120
Chronic liver diseases 235
Citrate 179
   buffer 234
Cleaning glasswares 18
Clostridium tetani 122
Clot retraction 180
   principle 180
   procedure 180
Coagulase test 118
   slide method 118
Coagulation time 173
Cocci 102
Colitis 225
Color reagent stock 221
Colorimeter 40
Colorimetric dinitrophenyl hydrazine
      method 237
Compound binocular microscope 35*f*
Continuous flow
   analysis 241
     disadvantages 241
   analyzer 241*f*
Corynebacterium minutissimum 59
Coverslip, cleaning of 11
COVID-19
   nitrile gloves, protocol for 258
   protocol for conducting 258
C-reactive protein 138
   principle 138
   procedure 139
   requirements 138
   test 135

Creatinine 222
Crenated red blood cells 78*f*
Crystal violet 17
   solution 17
Crystals cholesterol 81*f*
Culture media 112
Culture methods 117
Cuprous oxide 217
Cyanmethemoglobin method 153
   principle 153
   requirements 153
Cyst 130*f*
Cysteine 81*f*
   lactose electrolyte deficient medium 114
Cytoscope 112

D

Dark ground microscope 36, 36*f*
Diabetic curve 219
Diacetyl monoxime method 220
Diagnostic glucose values 220
Dichromate cleaning solution 11, 18
Differential leukocyte count 166, 167*f*
Dinitrophenyl hydrazine method 239
Diphtheria bacilli 103, 123
   culture 123
Dipotassium salt solution 18
Dirty glass slides, cleaning of 11
Discrete analyzer 242*f*
Disinfection 109
Disodium phenyl phosphate 233
Disposable boxes containing
   sputum 13
   stools 13
   urine 13
Distillation plant 61, 61*f*
   precautions 62
   procedure 62
   uses 62
Drabkin's solution 23
Drum-stick appearance 122
Dry cotton swab 156*f*
Dry heat 108
Duke's method 175
Dwarf tapeworm 135
   and egg 136*f*

E

Electric centrifuge 50
Electron microscope 38, 39*f*, 252
   construction 38
   uses 39

ELISA test 142, 144
   indirect 143
   sandwich 143
   uses of 143
Endoscope 112
Endotracheal tube 109
Enhanced glucose tolerance 220
Entamoeba
   coli 129
   histolytica 92, 129
Enteritis 225
Enterobius vermicularis 133
Enzymatic method 217
Enzyme 232
Eosinophil 169f
   cells 168
Epithelial cast 79, 80f
Epithelial cells 77
Erythrocyte 76, 148
   sedimentation rate 158
Esbach's albuminometer 70, 70f
   procedure 70
Exfoliative cytology 209
   uses 209
Exudative dermatosis 225

F

Fat, staining for 211
Fatty acids casts 79
Ferric chloride
   method of Henley 227
   solution of 18
Ferricyanide method 217
Fibrinogen 147
Fine granular casts 79
Fine needle aspiration cytology 202
   aspiration technique 203
   complications of 204
   contraindications of 203
   side effects of 204
   uses of 203
Fistulae 225
Food carbohydrates 215
Formalin-bicarbonate 22
Fouchet's reagent 18
Fouchet's test 75
Frozen section 207
Fungal infections, superficial 59
Fungal organisms causing diseases 128f

G

Germ containing material 14
   burial of 14, 14f

Giardia lamblia 130
Giemsa stain 16, 19
Glass pipettes, cleaning of 10
Glass rod and tube 152f
Glasswares
   cleaning of 10
   dirty 10
   new 10
Globulin 147
   qualitative tests for increase in 83
Glucose 74
   detection of 74
   tolerance test 218
      curve 219f
Gonococci 122
Gram iodine solution 19
Gram's iodine 106
Gram's staining 83, 92, 106, 127
   principle 106
   procedure 106
Grease-free coverslips, preparation of 11

H

Hand centrifuge 50
Hanging-drop preparation 104
Harris hematoxylin 205
Helminths 90f, 132
Hematological values 247
Hematology 145, 147
Hemoglobin
   estimation of 149, 185
   normal range of 155
Hemolytic disorders 178
Hemosiderin, stain for 210
Heparin 177
Hepatitis B surface antigen 144
Histopathological examination 195
Histopathological techniques 196
   fixation of specimen 196
   grossing of specimens 196
   labeling of tissues 197
   processing of tissue specimen 197
   reception of specimen 196
   registration 196
Histopathology 193, 195
Hookworm 132
   and eggs 133f
Hot air oven 47, 48f
   construction 47
   operation of 48
Human body fluids 67
Huyghens' eyepiece 31

Index

Hyaline cast 79
Hydatid cyst 203
Hydrochloric acid 19, 26, 27
Hydrogen sulfide test 119
Hymenolepis nana 135
Hypoxemia, severe 203

I

Ice-cream cup with lid 90f
Ideal blood smear 167f
Idiopathic exudative enteropathy 225
Immunology 135
Incineration 13
Incinerator 13f
    operating of 13
Indole test 119
Inoculum, primary 117
Inspissator 56, 56f
    construction 57
    operation 57
    precautions 57
    principle 56
    uses 57
Intact red blood cells 78f
Intact white blood cells 78f
Inulin fermentation 122
Iodine 236
    solution 236
Iris 32
Isotonic saline 22

J

Jaswant Singh and Bhattacharya stain 19

K

Kahn's antigen 142
Kahn's oscillator 142
Kahn's pipettes 142
Kahn's test 141
    principle 141
    procedure 142
Kahn's tube rack 142
Ketone bodies 75
Kidney
    cells from pelvis of 77
    tuberculosis of 74
Kovac's reagent 119

L

Laboratory
    arrangement of 6, 6f
    equipment 29
        microscope 29
    identification of bacteria 100
    infected material and clinical specimens, disposal of 13
    investigations 4
    requirements for 7
        chemicals 8
        furniture 7
        glassware 7
        instruments 7
        stationery 9
    technicians
        code of ethics for 3
        instructions for 5
    workers, avoiding infection of 101
Lag stage curve 220
Laminar airflow 46, 47
Lee and White method 174
    procedure 174
Leishman's stain 16, 20, 92, 168, 169f
    procedure of 168
Leprae bacilli 101
Leucine 81f
Leukemia 235
Leukocyte 77, 148
    count 82
        procedure of 168
    types of 168
Liquid media 113
    broth 113
    peptone water 113
    sugar media 113
Loeffler's serum 123
    slope 115
Löwenstein-Jensen medium 116
Lugol's iodine
    drop of 87
    solution 20
Lumbar puncture 82
Lungs, material of 89
Lupus erythematosus cell phenomenon 178
Lymph node metastasis 225
Lymphocyte
    cells 170
    large 169f
    small 169f

M

Macconkey's agar medium 118
Macconkey's media 117
Macconkey's medium 115

Malaria parasite, stages of 132f
Malarial parasites 131
Malloy and Evelyn method 229
Master mix, preparation of 259
Mattresses 110
Mean corpuscular
   hemoglobin 163
      concentration 163
   volume 162
Media, preparation of 113
Medical laboratory 1
Medical technician, responsibilities of 3
Meninges 100
Meningitis 82, 100
Methyl red test 119
Methylene blue 105
   aqueous 20
Microbiological safety cabinet 44f
Microbiology 97, 99
Microscope 29, 29f
   condenser 32, 32f
   construction 29
   eyepiece 32f
   interference 39
   magnification of 31
   mechanical adjustments 30
   mirror 32, 33f
   objectives 31f
   routine use of 34
   stand 30
Microscope optics 31
   aperture adjustment 33
   condenser 32f
      adjustment 33
      and iris 32
   drawtube 33
   eyepiece 31, 32f
   inclination 33
   light source 34f
   mechanical stage 34
   mirror 32, 33f
   objectives 31, 31f
   source of light 34
Microtome 199f
Moist heat 109
Molar solution 24
Monocyte 169f
   cells 170
Morphology 122
Muscular exercises 74
Museum specimens, organization of 202
Museum techniques 201
   fixation of specimen 201
   preparation of specimen 201
presentation of specimen 202
preservation of specimen 202
reception of specimen 201
restoration of specimen 202
Mycobacterium tuberculosis 123
Mycology 127

N

N sulfuric acid 144
Needles, cleaning of 11
Nephrotic syndrome 225
Neutralization reactions 136
Neutrophil 169f
   polymorphonuclear cells 168
N-glycosyl amine 215
Nitrate reduction test 120
Nonne-Apelt test 83
Normal fasting serum 216
Normal solution 24

O

Operation procedure 45
Optical density-cum-transmittance,
   measurement of 153
Optochin sensitivity test 122
Oral glucose tolerance test 220
Organic phosphate compounds 232
Ortho-toluidine
   method 215
   reagent 21, 215
Ovarian cyst 203
Oxalate 179
Oxaloacetate formed reacts 237
Oxidase test 120

P

Packed cell volume 161
   procedure 161
Paget's disease 235
Pandy's test 83
Papanicolaou's stain 83, 205
   eosin azure 36 206
   orange G6 205
   preparation 205
Paraffin wax, impregnation with 198
Parasitology 129
Peripheral blood film 169f
Perls stain 210
pH
   acidic 73
   alkaline 73

buffer solution 236
   normal 73
   phosphate buffer 237
   semen 94
Phase contrast microscope 35, 36f
Phenylalanine test 120
Pheochromocytoma 203
Phosphate buffer 239
Phosphotungstate reagent 231
Phosphotungstic acid 231
Photometer 40
   construction 40
   operation of 41
Picric acid 222
Pinworm 133
   and egg 134f
Plasma 147
   column of 162f
   glucose 216
Plasmodium
   falciparum 131
   malariae 131
   ovale 131
   vivax 131
Platelet 148
   thrombocytes 149f
Platelet count 172
   calculation 173
   procedure 173
   requirements 172
Pneumococci 122
Polarizing microscope 37, 37f
Polymerase chain reaction 62
   advantages of 65
   application of 64
   component of 63
   disadvantages 64
   machine 63f
   multiples 65
   nested 65
   principle 62
   results of 64
   reverse transcriptase 65
   run 259
   types of 64
Postrenal causes 222
Potassium 177
   ferricyanide 233
Precipitation reactions 136
Pregnancy test
   principle 140
   procedure 140
Prostate massage 235

Prostatic carcinoma 235
Prostatitis 203
Protein 74, 224
   detection of 74
   high 74
Proteinuria 225
Prothrombin 147
Prothrombin time 179
   increased 180
   principle 179
   procedure 179
Protozoa 88, 89f, 129
Pus
   cast 79, 80f
   cells 78f
Pyelonephritis 74

R

Random access analyzer 243
Rapid diagnosis, staining technique for 208
Rapid staining techniques 207
Reaction analysis 245
Reagent 15, 224
   handling 244
   preparation of 18, 258
Red blood cell 148, 149f
   count 159f
   total 155
   diluting fluid 21
   fragility of 178
   swollen 78f
Renal cause 222
Renal glycosuria 219
Reticulocyte count 170
Reticulum fibers 210
Rh blood grouping 188
Rh grouping
   slide test 188
   technique of 188
   tube test 188
Rheumatoid factor, latex fixation test for 137
Robertson's cooked meat media 116
Roundworm 133
   and eggs 133f
RT-PCR protocol 260

S

Safety cabinets, types of 43
Safranine solution 21
   stock 21
   working 21

Sahli's acid hematin method 149
Sahli's hemoglobinometer 152f
   consists 149
Sahli's pipette 152f
Saline
   eosin solution in 18
   normal 22, 224
Salmonella typhi 124
Sample
   dilutions of 26
   handling 243
   processing 243
Saturated sodium chloride solution 88
Scanning electron microscope 252, 256
   parts of 256
   working of 257
Schaudinn's solution 92
Semen
   collection of 93
   examination of 93
      microscopic 94
      physical 93
Sensing 245
Serological test 85
Serum 235
   aspartate transaminase 237, 239
   bilirubin 228
   uric acid, estimation of 230
Serum acid phosphatase 235
   estimation of 234
Serum alkaline phosphatase 233
   estimation of 232
Serum amylase 236
   estimation of 235
Serum glutamic
   oxaloacetic transaminase 237
   pyruvate transaminase 239
Shrunken white blood cells 78f
SI units 27
Silver nitrate titration method 84
   bacteriological examination 85
   principle 84
   procedures 84
   reagents 84
Single cell filter
   photo cell 41f
   photometer 40f
Skin scrapings 101
Slide, mounting tissue on 200
Smear
   examination of stained 92
   preparation 204

Sodium
   azide 224
   bicarbonate 233
   carbonate 231, 232
   chloride solution 22
   hydroxide 27, 222, 233
   thiosulfate aqueous solution 22
   tungstate 231
Solid media 114
Solution
   dilutions of 26
   preparation of 24
Somogyi method 235
Special staining methods 209
Specimen, bacterial contamination of 101
Sperm
   count 94
   diluting fluid 22
   morphology 95
   motility 94
Spermatozoa 77, 78f, 95f
   abnormal 95f
   normal 95f
Spirilla 104
Spirochetes 103
Sputum 100
   culture of 93
   examination of 89
      unstained 91
   microscopic examination 91
   physical examination 90
   reporting of 92
   smear, preparation of 91, 91f
   specimen, collection of 89
Squamous epithelial 78f
Squamous epithelial cells 77
Staining procedure 206
Staining solution 211
Staining technique 211
Standard acids and bases, preparation of 27
Standard creatinine stock 222
Starch solution 236
Sterilization 14, 108
   by boiling 15f
   chemical methods 109
   physical methods 108
Stock glucose solution 215
Stock phenol standard 233
Stock solution 171
Stock urea standard 221
Stool 100
   blood in 87
   collection of 86
      containers for 86f

Index

Stool examination 86
   bacteriological 88
   chemical 87
   microscopic 87
   physical 87
Streptococcus pyogenes 121
Studying fungi, methods for 127
Subnormal solution, preparation of 25
Sulfanilic acid 229
Sulfuric acid 26, 27
Syringe
   cleaning of 11
   parts of 12f

T

Taenia 135
   saginata 135
   solium 135
Tapeworm 135
   and egg 135f
Template addition protocol 259
Test tube test 119
Tetanus 99
Thermometers 111
Thrombocytes 148
Tissue specimen, embedding of 199
Toluidine blue method 207
Total leukocyte count 164, 165f
   procedure 165
   requirements 164
Total protein
   biuret method for 224
   estimation of 83, 224
Transmission electron microscope 252
   advantages 255
   applications 255
   disadvantages 255
   parts of 253
   sample preparation 255
   working principle of 254
Treponema pallidum 37, 125
Trichomonas 77, 78f
Trichuris trichiura 134
Triple phosphate 80, 81f
Triple sugar iron 120
Trisodium citrate 177
Trophozoites 130f
Tubercle bacilli 123
Tumor's cells 83
Tyrosine 81f

U

Urates 80
Uric acid 79, 81f, 230
   standard 231
Urinals 110
Urine 100
   blood in 76
   collection of 69
   color 71
   examination of 69
   odor 71
   pH of 73
   physical examination 71
   routine examination of 71
   sample 73
   specific gravity of 71, 72f
   specimen, preservation of 70
   volume 71
Urinometer 71, 72
   bile pigments 75
   chemical examination 74
   construction 72
   microscopic examination 76
   procedure 73

V

van Gieson's stain 209, 211
   procedure 209
   requirement 209
Vascular lesions 203
Venereal disease research laboratory test 140
Venous blood 175
Verhoeff's elastic stain 212
Vertical autoclave 42f
Vibrio 103
   cholerae 88, 124
Voges-Proskauer test 121

W

Water bath 59, 60f, 142
   construction 59
   operation 60
   precautions 60
   uses 60
Water
   bacteriological examination of 125, 126f
   collection of 125
Water sample
   dispatching of 125
   packing of 125

Waxed cardboard 86f
Westergren ESR pipettes stand 161f
Westergren method 160
    procedure 160
    requirements 160
Westergren pipette 161f
Whipworm 134
    and egg 134f
White apron 12
White blood cell 148, 149f
    diluting fluid 22
White coat, uses of 12
Widal test 135, 136
    principle 136
    procedure 137
Wilder's silver impregnation method 210
Willis solution 22
Wintrobe method 159
    procedure 159
    uses 159
Wintrobe's ESR tube 160f
Wintrobe's hematocrit tube 161

Wintrobe's tube, graduation on 160f
Wireloop 117f
    stand for 117f
Wood's lamp 57, 58f
    applications of 59
    examination, technique of 58
Working acid reagent 220
Working color reagent 221
Working creatinine standard 223

Y

Yeast 77
    cells 78f

Z

Ziehl-Neelsen stain 16, 21, 92, 107
    modified 15, 17
    principle 107
    procedure 107
    smears 83
    solution for 20

EU GSPR Authorised Reprsentative
Logos Europe, 9 rue Nicolas Poussin
1700, La Rochelle, France
Phone: +33 (0) 6 67 93 73 78
E-mail: contact@logoseurope.eu

www.ingramcontent.com/pod-product-compliance
Ingram Content Group UK Ltd.
Pitfield, Milton Keynes, MK11 3LW, UK
UKHW021832140426
5217IPUK00021B/1400